Self-assessment cases in surgical imaging

by

Chris J. Harvey

Consultant Radiologist, Hammersmith Hospital, London, UK

Hugh R.S. Roberts

Consultant Radiologist, Christchurch Hospital, Christchurch, New Zealand

Nigel Davies

Consultant Radiologist, Worthing Hospital, Worthing, UK

Nicola H. Strickland

Consultant Radiologist, Hammersmith Hospital, London, UK

and

John H. Scurr

Honorary Consultant Surgeon and Senior Lecturer, Middlesex and University College Hospitals, London, UK

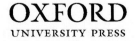

OXFORD
UNIVERSITY PRESS

*This book has been printed digitally and produced in a standard specification
in order to ensure its continuing availability*

OXFORD
UNIVERSITY PRESS

Great Clarendon Street, Oxford OX2 6DP

Oxford University Press is a department of the University of Oxford.
It furthers the University's objective of excellence in research, scholarship,
and education by publishing worldwide in

Oxford New York

Auckland   Cape Town Dar es Salaam Hong Kong Karachi
Kuala Lumpur Madrid Melbourne Mexico City   Nairobi
New Delhi Shanghai Taipei Toronto
With offices in
Argentina Austria Brazil Chile Czech Republic France Greece
Guatemala Hungary Italy Japan South Korea Poland Portugal
Singapore Switzerland Thailand Turkey Ukraine Vietnam

Oxford is a registered trade mark of Oxford University Press
in the UK and in certain other countries

Published in the United States
by Oxford University Press Inc., New York

© Oxford University Press, 2005

ISBN 978-0-19-263164-0

Printed and bound by CPI Antony Rowe, Eastbourne

Foreword

It is a long time since I last read a book from cover to cover and enjoyed every page. High quality images combined with outstanding clinical reviews of the conditions covered makes this a superb teaching resource for undergraduates and postgraduates alike.

With the hours available for formal training being eroded, this book provides an ideal substitute and should be essential reading for those taking intercollegiate MRCS. Even those who are already specializing will find the images and commentary related to cases seen in their specialty of great value.

Mr Gordon Williams
Consultant Urologist
and Chairman
Joint Committee on
Higher Surgical Training (UK)
Hammersmith Hospital
London, UK

Preface

This book has been produced in response to a perceived need by candidates approaching their MRCS examination for guidance in radiological diagnosis and investigation of common surgical problems. Radiology occupies a central role in patient management and therefore it is essential that candidates have a sound knowledge of imaging techniques and interpretation, both for examinations and for their future careers. As well as the traditional imaging modalities the newer techniques such as computed tomography (CT), magnetic resonance (MR), ultrasound, nuclear medicine, and interventional radiology are amply covered. For each case the answer includes explanation of the radiographic appearances as well as discussion of the radiological investigation of the condition. The cases discussed cover the majority of the material likely to be encountered in the MRCS and final medical examinations.

It is anticipated that this book will be primarily aimed at surgical specialist registrars (SpRs) facing the MRCS, but will also be of value to medical SpRs, medical students, preregistration house officers, radiology SpRs, and established clinicians who wish to refresh their knowledge in radiology.

London   C.J.H.
2004   H.R.S.R.
                                                                                                       N.D.
                                                                                                       N.H.S.
                                                                                                       J.H.S.

Acknowledgements

The authors would like to thank Dr James Pilcher, Dr Nandita De Souza, Ms Louise Farmer, Dr Josh Hollway, Dr Alison Graham, Prof David Cosgrove, Ms Cliona Cunningham, Mr Tony McArthur, Dr Paul Tait, Dr Alissa Connors, and Dr James Hodson who generously donated radiographs, read manuscripts, and gave encouragement during the preparation of this book.

Contents

Abbreviations

5-HIAA	5-hydroxyindoleacetic acid
AAA	abdominal aortic aneurysm
ACAS	Asymptomatic Carotid Atherosclerosis Study
ACL	anterior cruciate ligament
ACTH	adenocorticotrophic hormone
ALARA (principle)	as low as reasonably achievable (radiation dose)
AML	renal angiomyolipoma
AP	anteroposterior
APACHE	Acute Physiology and Chronic Health Enquiry (score)
APC	adenomatous polyposis
APUD	amine precursor uptake and decarboxylation (system)
ARDS	adult respiratory distress syndrome
AXR	abdominal X-ray
CAPD	continuous ambulatory peritoneal dialysis
CCA	common carotid artery
CF	cystic fibrosis
CFA	common femoral artery
COPD	chronic obstructive pulmonary disease
CPA	cerebellopontine angle
CSF	cerebrospinal fluid
CT	computed tomography
CTPA	CT pulmonary angiogram
CXR	chest X-ray
DCIS	ductal carcinoma *in situ*
DJ	duodeno-jejunal
DVT	deep vein thrombosis
ECA	external carotid artery
ECST	European Carotid Surgery Trial
EDV	end-diastolic velocity
ERCP	endoscopic retrograde cholangiopancreatography
ETT	endotracheal tube
EVAR	endovascular aneurysm repair
^{18}FDG	18-fluorodeoxyglucose
FSH	follicle stimulating hormone
GH	growth hormone
GIST	gastrointestinal stromal tumour
GORD	gastro-oesophageal reflux disease
HSG	hysterosalpinography
HU	hounsfield units

I^{131} MIBG	I^{131} labelled metaiodobenzylguanidine
ICA	internal carotid artery
IMT	intima-media thickness
IR(ME)R	Ionizing Radiation (Medical Exposure) Regulations
IV	intravenous
IVC	inferior vena cava
IVU	intravenous urography
LES	lower oesophageal sphincter
LH	luteinizing hormone
MR	magnetic resonance
MRCP	magnetic resonance cholangiopancreatogram
MRI	MR imaging
MUCG	micturating cystourethrogram
NASCET	North American Symptomatic Carotid Endarterectomy Trial
NF	neurofibromatosis
PA	posteroanterior
PAVM	pulmonary arteriovenous malformation
PC	pelvicalyceal
PDA	patent ductus arteriosus
PE	pulmonary embolism
PET	positron emission tomography
PSC	primary sclerosing cholangitis
PSV	peak systolic velocity
PTA	percutaneous transluminal angioplasty
PTH	parathormone
RCC	renal cell carcinoma
ROI	region of interest
SCFE	slipped capital femoral epiphysis
SFA	superficial femoral artery
SFV	superficial femoral vein
SMA	superior mesenteric artery
SMV	superior mesenteric vein
Sv	sievert
TB	tuberculosis
TIA	transient ischaemic attack
TM	testicular microlithiasis
TOF	tracheo-oesophageal fistula
TS	tuberous sclerosis
TSH	thyroid stimulating hormone
UC	ulcerative colitis
US	ultrasound
UTI	urinary tract infection
VHL	Von Hippel–Lindau (disease)

VSD	ventricular septal defect
V/Q	ventilation/perfusion (scan)
VUJ	vesicoureteric junction

Introduction and guidance on interpretation of imaging modalities

The specialty of diagnostic radiology encompasses a wide spectrum of imaging modalities that can be used to provide the clinician with enough information to make a diagnosis. Diagnostic imaging includes plain film radiography, contrast-enhanced radiography, ultrasound, computed tomography (CT), magnetic resonance (MR), nuclear medicine, and interventional radiology.

X-rays were discovered just over a century ago by Roentgen and are used in all forms of plain film and contrast-enhanced radiography, interventional radiology, and CT. They lie at the high-energy end of the electromagnetic spectrum and are produced by passing a high voltage across two terminals in a vacuum tube, causing high-energy electrons to be emitted from a cathode; these electrons then bombard the anode. The resultant interaction of electrons produces X-rays. A brief introduction to each modality and its interpretation is necessary to help the reader understand how these modalities are used in clinical problem-solving.

Imaging modalities

Plain film radiography

At the energies used in diagnostic imaging different tissues will appear more or less transparent to X-rays. The resultant shadows can be detected using various means such as intensifying screen/photographic film combinations or fluoroscopic systems. The most common technique for imaging an X-ray is to expose a single image on a film sandwiched between two fluorescent screens that convert X-rays to visible light in a cassette. Real-time fluoroscopy is also possible using image intensifiers and television systems.

Different tissues produce different degrees of X-ray attenuation, basically reflecting their density, thickness, and atomic number. Air, such as that in the lungs, is transparent to X-rays and therefore appears black (since a high dose of relatively unattenuated X-rays is hitting the radiographic film and exposing it by reducing the ionic silver halide in it to high concentrations of black elemental silver). Most soft tissues are of intermediate 'greyness', while calcified tissues, such as bone, appear white (since their high tissue density markedly attenuates the X-ray beam so that a relatively low dose of X-rays gets through to expose the radiographic film). When there is a large difference in either density or atomic number between two adjacent organs, then the contours of these structures will be clearly visualized on a radiograph because of the high inherent natural contrast (e.g. heart and lungs, bone, and soft tissue).

On a conventional radiograph, four basic densities can be resolved: air; fat; soft tissues; and calcified tissues. An example of the value of natural contrast is the loss of silhouette sign. On a normal chest radiograph the heart and mediastinal interface is clearly visualized against the black lungs. However, in the presence of adjacent lung collapse or consolidation, more X-rays are absorbed by the diseased lung, rendering it more opaque and of similar X-ray attenuating density to the adjacent mediastinum, resulting in loss of the contour of adjacent structures (loss of the silhouette sign). An example of loss of the silhouette sign occurs in left lower lobe collapse: the medial aspect of the left hemidiaphragm and the lateral border of the lower descending thoracic aorta is lost because these structures now lie adjacent to the collapsed left lower lobe, which is denser than the alveolar air that would be present in a normal left lower lobe.

Contrast agents

When there is no natural contrast, contrast agents are used to artificially alter X-ray attenuation locally (e.g. blood vessels in an organ). Contrast media may be divided into 'positive' contrast agents of high radiodensity (e.g. iodine, barium) and 'negative' agents of low density (e.g. air, carbon dioxide). Iodine and barium block X-rays and appear white, while gas (air or carbon dioxide) appears black. Double contrast combinations of air and barium can also be used in many situations to opacify body compartments.

Contrast media may be used to demonstrate structural abnormalities (e.g. colon cancer in double contrast barium enema) or to derive functional information (e.g. delayed opacification of the renal tract due to obstruction in intravenous urography (IVU)). Contrast agents have a wide spectrum of applications and may be introduced orally, by cannulation of orifices (e.g. hysterosalpinography (HSG)), via tubes (e.g. T-tube cholangiography), intravenously, or percutaneously.

Interpretation of the chest radiograph

- **Technical factors**. A posteroanterior (PA) chest radiograph is taken with the X-ray tube behind the patient and the cassette (or detector) against the anterior chest. The medial ends of the clavicles should be equidistant from the spinous processes in a correctly centred film.
- **Trachea**. This should normally be central. It may be deviated away from a superior mediastinal mass, e.g. thyroid goitre, or pulled by any process that causes volume loss, e.g. lung fibrosis.
- **Heart**. The normal cardiothoracic ratio (ratio of transverse cardiac diameter to transverse inner thoracic diameter) is less than 50%. The entire border of the heart and mediastinum should be clearly visualized.
- **Hilar regions**. These are made up of the pulmonary arteries and veins (predominantly the upper lobe pulmonary vein and the lower lobe pulmonary artery). They have a concave lateral margin. They are of equal density and the right hilum is lower than the left.
- **Lungs**. These should be equal in density. When there is asymmetry, the side of decreased vascularity is usually the abnormal side. Inspect for focal lesions.
- **Diaphragms**. On full inspiration the right hemidiaphragm is at the level of the sixth rib anteriorly. Inspect for free subdiaphragmatic gas due to perforation of a viscus (unless there is a known iatrogenic cause, such as a recent laparotomy or continuous ambulatory

peritoneal dialysis (CAPD)). Also look for subphrenic abscesses, calcified liver lesions, gallstones, and dilated bowel loops.

- **Review areas**. Check that both breasts are present; look for lesions behind the heart silhouette and lung apices, or at the hila. Check the bones for focal abnormalities and density, and check the shoulder joints if they are visible on the chest radiograph. Check the skin for surgical emphysema or calcified parasites.

Interpretation of the abdominal radiograph

- **Calcifications**. Inspect for renal tract calculi, gallstones, pancreatic calcification, appendoliths, and calcified aortic aneurysms. Most calcifications are not significant (phleboliths, lymph nodes, arterial walls, fibroids, and costal cartilage).
- **Bowel gas pattern**. Gas is normally seen in the stomach and colon. Small amounts may be seen in the small bowel. Colonic calibre is variable but a transverse colonic diameter of 5.5 cm is taken as the upper limit of normal. Dilatation of the bowel occurs in obstruction, paralytic ileus, ischaemia, and inflammatory bowel disease. Inspect for free intraperitoneal gas, which may be recognized as Rigler's sign with visualization of both the inner and outer bowel wall. Look for intramural gas.
- **Ectopic gas**. Look for pneumobilia, portal venous gas, and gas in the genitourinary tract.
- **Viscera**. The liver, spleen, kidneys, and psoas silhouettes may normally be seen.
- **Pelvic masses**. These may be bladder or gynaecological lesions.

Interpretation of the intravenous urogram (IVU)

On the plain film identify renal tract calcification: calculi; nephrocalcinosis; prostatic calcification; tuberculosis (TB); and tumours.

The **IVU film series** should be inspected for the following.

- Renal length is equal to that of about three lumbar vertebrae. The left kidney is slightly larger and higher than the right.
- The renal outline should be smooth; any indentations or bulges warrant further investigation. Patients with renal masses may have associated calyceal distortion.
- Calyceal dilatation may be caused by obstruction or by disease of the papilla (e.g. papillary necrosis, pyelonephritis, reflux nephropathy).
- The renal pelves are inspected for filling defects (e.g. tumour, stones, blood clot, sloughed papilla).
- Ureters. Opacification of the whole ureter suggests distal obstruction. Displacement occurs in retroperitoneal pathology (e.g. retroperitoneal fibrosis causes medial displacement).
- Bladder contour should be smooth and no post-micturition residual volume should be seen.

Interpretation of barium studies

- **Barium swallow and meal**. The oesophagus should have a smooth mucosa with no dilatation. Normal oesophageal impressions may be due to cricopharyngeus muscle and the posterior venous plexus in the cervical region, aortic arch, left main bronchus, and left atrium.

- **Small bowel studies**. A bowel diameter of 3 cm is taken as the upper limit of normal. Strictures may be benign (smooth tapering edge) or malignant (short with overhanging edges, termed 'shouldering'). The same rule applies to the colon. Normal bowel fold thickness is less than 2 mm. Folds may be thickened in malabsorption, oedema, infiltrative diseases, and inflammatory bowel disease.
- **Colonic studies**. Contrast enemas should be analysed for strictures (benign and malignant). Displacement of small and large bowel loops due to extrinsic masses, e.g. abscesses, pancreatic lesions, and renal lesions.

Computed tomography (CT)

CT uses X-rays to construct axial images. Patients receive a considerable dose of ionizing radiation, but excellent anatomical information is obtained. Using fast modern spiral and multidetector CT the whole body can be scanned in 20–40 seconds, fast enough to allow acquisition of different phases of contrast enhancement (e.g. arterial phase and portal venous phase). Three-dimensional, multiplanar, and angiographic imaging is routine. Tissues absorb X-rays by differing amounts; this is referred to as attenuation. Lesions of high attenuation are white (fresh haemorrhage, calcification) and low attenuation lesions are black (air, fat). The amount of absorption, with reference to water, is measured in hounsfield units (HU; after Sir Geoffrey Hounsfield, the inventor of CT). Thus water has a HU of zero, air –1000 HU, fat –100 to –60 HU, soft tissues +40 to 60 HU, and calcium +400 to 1000 HU, approximately.

CT characterization of an undiagnosed lesion gives information regarding its composition and degree of enhancement with contrast agent.

Radiation dosage

X-rays cause tissue ionization resulting in liberation of electrons and the production of an ion pair, which can lead to potentially harmful physicochemical effects, including the production of free radicals that potentially may lead to both carcinogenesis and mutagenesis.

It is extremely important that the radiation dose both to patients and to medical personnel is minimized. X-ray exposure should be avoided unless it produces a net benefit to the patient, and that exposure should be kept as low as reasonably achievable (the ALARA principle). The Ionizing Radiation (Medical Exposure) Regulations (IR(ME)R) introduced by the UK Department of Health in May 2000 require that all medical exposures to ionizing radiation are clinically justified and authorized.

The biological damage produced by a given exposure can be calculated by summing the absorbed radiation dose to individual organs weighted for their radiation sensitivity. This value (the effective dose equivalent) is measured in milliSieverts (mSv), and gives an estimate of the adverse effects of different types of radiological procedures. The average background radiation exposure in the UK is 2.5 mSv/year. The dose from a chest X-ray is very low (comparable to that experienced from cosmic radiation during a London to Paris flight) while the dose from procedures such as CT may be hundreds of times higher (Table 1).

Table 1 Effective dose from radiological procedures (approximate figures)

	Effective dose (mSv)	Relative dose	Equivalent period of background dose
Chest X-ray (single PA film)	0.02	1	3 days
Abdominal X-ray (single)	1	50	6 months
Lumbar spine series	1.3	65	7 months
Intravenous urography	2.5	125	14 months
Barium enema	7	350	3 years
CT abdomen/pelvis	10	500	4.5 years

Ultrasound

Ultrasound produces real-time, two-dimensional images of body structures using sound waves, is non-invasive, quick, and inexpensive, and avoids the use of ionizing radiation.

The image is derived from reflected sound waves at boundaries of differing acoustic impedance. Bright (echogenic) lesions equate with good reflectors such as calcium and air where a posterior acoustic shadow may be seen. Fluid is black (anechoic) as it transmits sound well. The real-time nature of ultrasonography is highly suited to renal biopsy and to other interventional procedures.

Doppler ultrasonography is based on the principle that, when incident sound waves are reflected from a moving structure, the frequency is shifted by an amount proportional to the velocity of the reflector (e.g. a red blood cell flowing in a vessel). This shift can be quantified and displayed as a spectral Doppler scan or a colour overlay (colour Doppler). Flow towards the probe is conventionally displayed as red and flow away as blue. Using colour Doppler, vessel patency, direction of flow, and abnormal vascularity can be determined. Spectral Doppler examination of a vessel gives time-dependent velocities that are useful in assessing vascular stenoses.

Magnetic resonance (MR)

MR imaging (MRI) is based on the fact that protons spin and have an associated magnetic field. When an external radiofrequency pulse is delivered, protons resonate (energy is transferred to the protons). When the pulse is switched off, the acquired magnetization decays and the time-decay curve is characteristic of tissue types and thus pathological processes. The images acquired may be T1- or T2-weighted. On a T1-weighted image fat typically gives a high signal and on T2 images water (urine, bile, cerebrospinal fluid (CSF), etc.) is bright (white). The addition of fat suppression (removing the signal from fat) causes the fat to become black (e.g. Short TI Inversion Recovery (STIR) sequence). MR does not use ionizing radiation but is expensive. There are no known biological hazards of MR. Pacemakers, hearing aids, many metal clips, and prosthetic valves are contraindicated in MR scanners because of their potential movement in the magnetic field. The most commonly used intravenous (IV) MR contrast agents are gadolinium chelates, which enhance signal on T1 sequences.

Nuclear medicine

Unlike other imaging modalities, nuclear medicine provides functional rather than anatomical information. It is based on the imaging of radionuclide-labelled molecules that are taken up physiologically by different body organs. The most widely used radioisotope is technetium-99m, which emits gamma rays that are detected by gamma cameras.

Positron emission tomography (PET) scanning uses cyclotron-produced isotopes (particularly the glucose analogue, 18-fluorodeoxyglucose (^{18}FDG)) of extremely short half-life that emit positrons. PET scanning can be used to document the biodistribution and fate of key molecules in metabolic pathways. It is particularly useful in looking for tumour activity as glucose is avidly metabolized compared with normal tissue. It is used to differentiate benign from malignant pulmonary nodules, recurrent or residual brain tumour, and postradiation therapy change from recurrent malignancy. It is also useful in the follow-up of tumours to look for small metastases and in distinguishing benign from malignant lymphadenopathy.

Question 1

This 8-month-old infant presented with colicky abdominal pain and bloody stools. What are the radiological findings on this supine abdominal film (Fig. 1a)? What is the diagnosis?

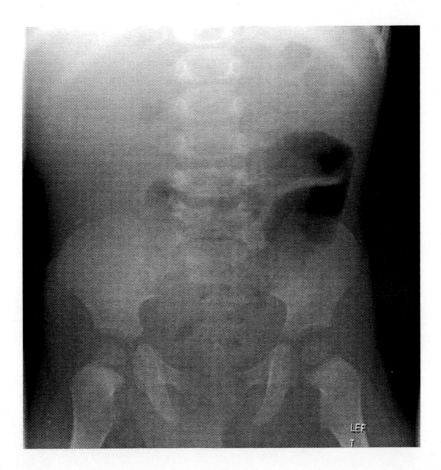

Fig. 1a

Answer 1: Intussusception

Findings: The supine abdominal radiograph shows an absence of bowel gas in the right iliac fossa. There is a soft tissue mass in the epigastrium consistent with an intussuscepted caecum/ ascending colon. There is no free intraperitoneal gas or evidence of small bowel obstruction.

Intussusception is one of the most common abdominal emergencies of early childhood. It is most commonly ileocolic (75–95%) in children compared with ileo-ileal (40%) in adults. The aetiology is idiopathic in over 95% in children and is thought to be due to lymphoid hyperplasia of Peyer's patches and mesenteric adenitis. A lead point is identified in 5% of cases (Meckel's diverticulum, enteric cyst/polyp, appendiceal inflammation, Henoch–Schonlein purpura, or inspissated meconium).

Only 5% of cases of intussusception are seen in adults. Of these cases, 20% are idiopathic. The remaining 80% show a specific cause, including benign neoplasm (one-third), malignant neoplasm (one-fifth), Meckel's diverticulum, foreign body, and trauma.

The diagnosis often requires a high level of suspicion. The plain radiograph is normal in 25%, but shows an abdominal soft tissue mass in 50% (commonly in the right upper quadrant). Features of small bowel obstruction are present in 25%. Barium studies can be used in

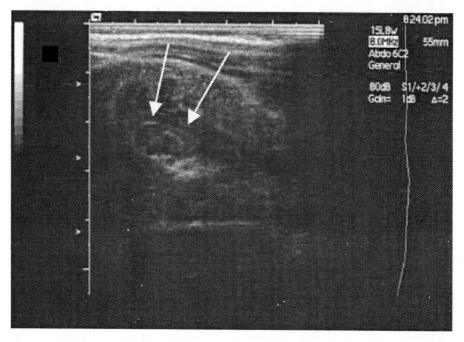

Fig. 1b   Ultrasound shows a bowel mass with concentric layers consisting of an interssusceptum (arrows) within the intussuscipiens.

diagnosis, but have limitations when compared with ultrasound (Fig. 1b), which is up to 100% sensitive. Ultrasound demonstrates the concentric rings of the different layers of the intussusception (referred to as doughnut/target/bulls-eye/pseudo-kidney) with vessels seen entering the mass on colour Doppler. CT (Fig 1c) also shows multiple concentric rings and may make the proximal obstruction easier to appreciate. CT may also demonstrate the cause.

In children, intussusception may be managed by pneumatic or hydrostatic (barium) reduction under ultrasound or fluoroscopic guidance. Absolute contraindications to these procedures are peritonitis, shock, or perforation. A paediatric surgeon should be informed and available prior to attempted reduction. Success rates of greater than 90% are reported with 0.4% incidence of perforation and a recurrence rate of 3.5–10% within 48 hours. Intussusceptions that have been symptomatic for longer than 48 hours are less likely to be reduced. Surgery is usually required in adult intussusception. It allows reduction of the intussusception and identification of any causative lesion.

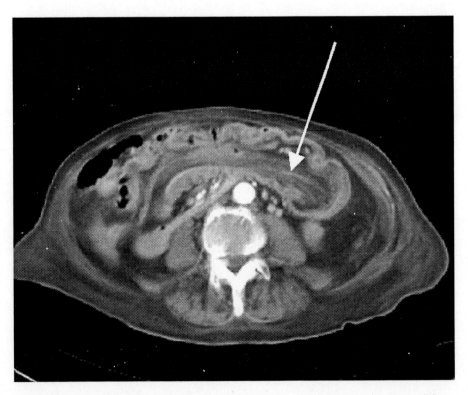

Fig. 1c   CT of an adult intussusception with mesenteric fat and vessels (arrow) in the lumen of the transverse colon.

Question 2

This 8-week-old boy presented with copious vomiting. An ultrasound of the abdomen (Fig. 2a) revealed this abnormality in the epigastrium. What is the diagnosis?

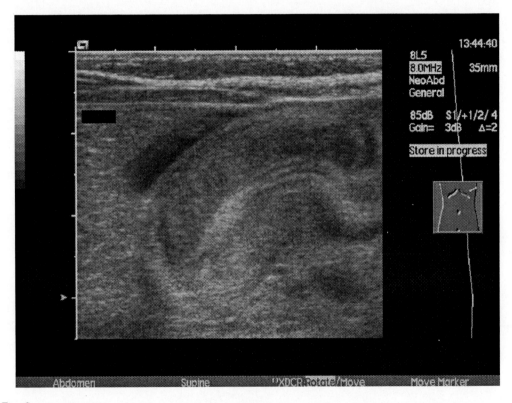

Fig. 2a

Answer 2: Hypertrophic pyloric stenosis

Findings: The pyloric canal is elongated (2.39 cm; Fig. 2b). The muscular wall is thickened (0.53 cm; Fig. 2b) around the central echogenic mucosa.

Hypertrophic pyloric stenosis usually presents at 2–8 weeks with non-bilious projectile vomiting, has a male preponderance (M:F 4–5:1) with a dominant polygenic trait, and is more common in full-term infants compared with the premature. The diagnosis may be made clinically when an olive-shaped pyloric mass is palpable to the right of the epigastrium. Ultrasound is the investigation of choice with a barium meal seldom necessary except in equivocal cases or when there is insufficient paediatric ultrasound expertise. The ultrasound criteria are: an elongated pyloric canal (≥ 17 mm); a transverse pyloric diameter of ≥ 13 mm; and a pyloric muscular wall thickness of ≥ 3 mm. The real-time nature of ultrasound allows the operator to look for failure of propagation of peristaltic waves into the duodenum when gastric contractions reach the pylorus, associated with failure of gastric emptying. This sign, in conjunction with pyloric muscular enlargement, increases diagnostic confidence.

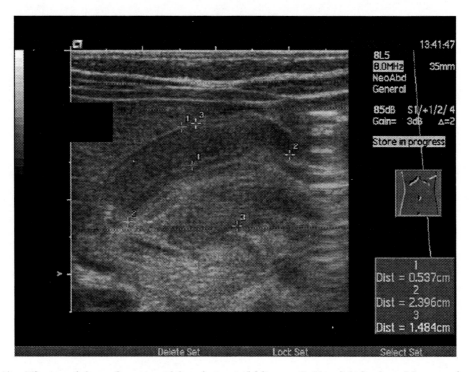

Fig. 2b   Ultrasound shows elongation of the pyloric canal (distance 2–2) and thickening of the muscular wall (distance 1–1) in this case of hypertrophic pyloric stenosis.

Question 3

This 56-year-old lady presented with dysphagia. A barium swallow was performed (Fig. 3). What is the diagnosis? Give two complications.

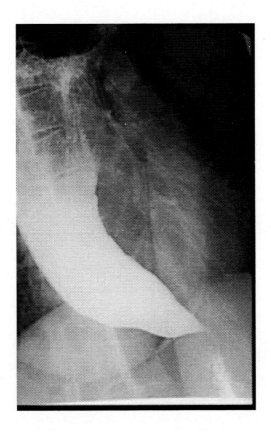

Fig. 3

Answer 3: Achalasia

Potential complications

1   Aspiration;
2   Carcinoma of the oesophagus.

Findings: The barium swallow shows a markedly dilated oesophagus with food residue. There is a 'bird beak' appearance of the distal oesophagus.

Achalasia is characterized by failure of relaxation of the lower oesophageal sphincter resulting in proximal dilatation and there is also loss of peristaltic contractions. A decrease in the number of ganglionic cells is seen in the nerve plexus of the oesophageal wall. Chagas' disease produces a similar clinical picture.

Patients usually have dysphagia for both solids and liquids and pain may be a prominent feature. The diagnosis is made by barium swallow and manometry.

The barium swallow shows oesophageal dilatation. No primary peristaltic waves pass beyond the upper thoracic oesophagus. Contrast studies classically show a smooth tapering 'bird-beak' or 'rat's tail' appearance of the distal oesophagus with small quantities of contrast intermittently squirting into the stomach. Achalasia must be differentiated from scleroderma and a distal oesophageal carcinoma. In scleroderma the oesophagus is usually less dilated and free gastro-oesophageal reflux is present which may result in benign peptic oesophageal stricture mimicking achalasia. Less dilatation is present with an oesophageal carcinoma, and the stricture is frequently irregular and asymmetrical. Oesophagoscopy should be performed to exclude a secondary malignancy. Treatment is via balloon dilatation or surgical intervention (myotomy).

Question 4

This 36-year-old man presented with 6 hours of central abdominal pain. An abdominal radiograph (Fig. 4a) and ultrasound (Fig. 4b) were performed. What abnormalities are present? What is the diagnosis?

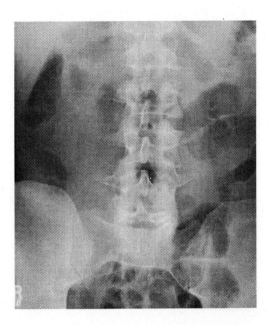

Fig. 4a

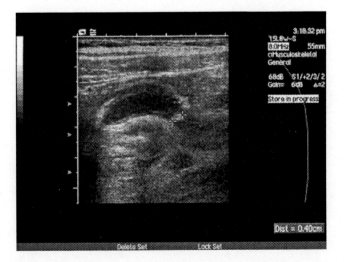

Fig. 4b

Answer 4: Acute appendicitis

Findings: The abdominal radiograph shows a calcified faecolith in the appendix (appendolith) in the right iliac fossa with some dilated loops of small bowel consistent with an associated ileus. The ultrasound revealed a thickened dilated appendix with an appendolith (between measuring callipers).

The combination of an appendolith and abdominal pain equates with a 90% probability of acute appendicitis. An appendolith in acute appendicitis has a high probability of gangrene/perforation. An ultrasound or CT is therefore useful to exclude an abscess.

Plain abdominal film findings in acute appendicitis:

- Calcified appendolith, 7–15%;
- Caecal ileus (gas fluid level in gangrene);
- Small bowel ileus;
- Extraluminal gas (in 33% of perforations). Pneumoperitoneum is rare;
- Colon cut-off sign (amputation of gas at the hepatic flexure) due to spastic ascending colon.

Ultrasound criteria:

- Sensitivity, 77–94%; specificity, 90%; accuracy, 90–95%;
- Visualization of a non-compressible aperistaltic distended appendix. The normal appendix is seen in 2% of adults and 50% of children;
- Thickened echo-poor wall of > 2 mm and total transverse diameter of > 6 mm;
- Localized periappendiceal fluid;
- Prominent echogenic mesoappendiceal/caecal fat (indicative of inflammation);
- Increased Doppler blood flow seen in and around the appendix;

CT features:

- Circumferential thickening of appendix wall;
- Diameter of appendix > 6 mm;
- Periappendiceal collections/abscess;
- Periappendiceal fat/mesenteric inflammatory change;
- CT allows diagnosis of retrocaecal appendicitis (Fig. 4c) which will be missed on ultrasound.

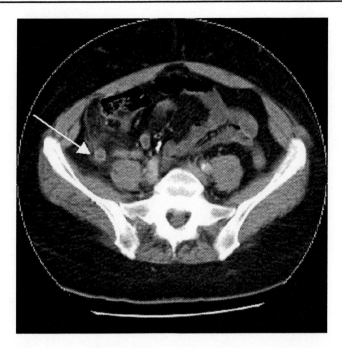

Fig. 4c   Contrast-enhanced CT section showing retrocaecal appendicitis (arrow) with adjacent streaky inflammatory change.

Question 5

This 24-hour-old term neonate presented with abdominal distension and vomiting with absolute constipation. A plain abdominal radiograph (Fig. 5a) and a gastrografin enema (Fig. 5b) are shown. What is the diagnosis?

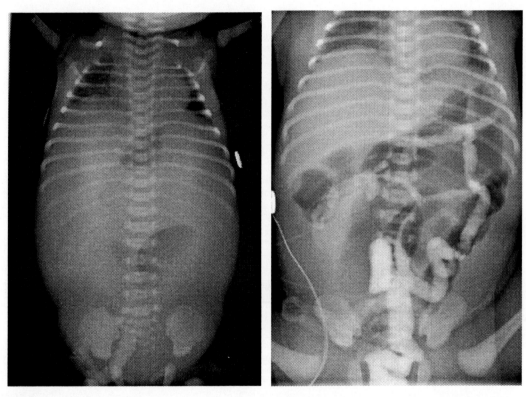

Fig. 5a   Fig. 5b

Answer 5: Meconium peritonitis; ileal atresia

Findings: The plain radiograph shows speckled calcification over the right flank consistent with meconium peritonitis. The contrast enema demonstrates a small calibre colon (microcolon). The contrast stops at the site of the meconium peritonitis. The small bowel is dilated consistent with obstruction.

Meconium peritonitis is due to a sterile chemical peritonitis secondary to perforation of bowel proximal to a high grade/complete obstruction that reseals *in utero*. Peritoneal calcification then ensues.

Causes of meconium peritonitis:

- Atresia (secondary to an ischaemic event 50%) of: (1) small bowel (usually jejunum or ileum) or (2) colon (uncommon);
- Bowel obstruction (46%) due to: (1) meconium ileus; (2) volvulus, hernia; or (3) intussusception, congenital bands, Meckel's diverticulum.

Causes of a microcolon:

- Meconium ileus. This is a distal small bowel obstruction secondary to inspissated meconium that impacts in the ileum. Usually due to cystic fibrosis (CF; almost 100%) but only 10–15% of infants with CF present with meconium ileus;
- Small bowel atresia;
- Hirschsprung's disease (long segment);
- Meconium plug syndrome (functional immaturity of the colon seen in neonates of diabetic mothers).

A gastrografin enema can be therapeutic as well as diagnostic in meconium ileus and meconium plug syndrome since the hyperosmolar contrast has hygroscopic and osmotic effects facilitating the passage of meconium.

Question 6

This neonate had failed to pass meconium in the first 24 hours since birth. A contrast enema was performed (Fig. 6). What is the diagnosis?

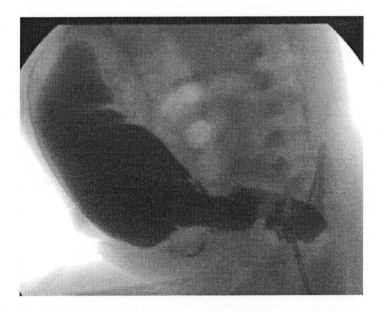

Fig. 6

Answer 6: Hirschsprung's disease

Findings: The rectum is narrowed with a short transition between the proximal dilated sigmoid and the narrowed rectum.

Hirshsprung's disease is characterized by an absence of parasympathetic ganglia in muscle and submucosal layers secondary to an arrest of craniocaudal migration of neuroblasts along vagal trunks *in utero*. This leads to failure of relaxation in the aganglionic segment and therefore impairment of peristalsis.

The incidence is 1 in 5000, familial in 4%, more common in males (4–9:1, M:F) and is rarely seen in premature infants. The condition commonly presents in the first 6 weeks of life with failure to pass meconium or constipation, vomiting, and abdominal distension.

The aganglionic segment is seen as a hypertonic narrowing and always extends proximally from the anus. The transition point is most commonly sited in the rectosigmoid (80%), so-called short segment disease, but extends more proximally in 15% (long segment disease). Total colonic aganglionosis occurs in 5% and, very rarely, sparing of the rectum occurs with skip aganglionosis.

The diagnosis is made by contrast enema. This identifies the transition site and the length of the aganglionic segment and excludes other causes of obstruction. Digital rectal examination and cleansing enema should be avoided prior to the contrast enema because they may dilate the distal narrowed segment thus obscuring the transition zone. The diagnosis is confirmed by suction rectal biopsies. Uncommon complications include necrotizing enterocolitis and colon perforation.

Question 7

This neonate presented with coughing during feeding. An oesophagogram was performed (Fig. 7a). What does this demonstrate? What other investigations should be performed?

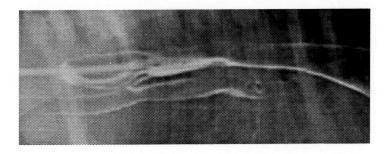

Fig. 7a

Answer 7: Tracheo-oesophageal fistula (TOF)

A renal ultrasound and a spinal survey are indicated to look for associated abnormalities.

Findings: The study should be performed with the baby in the prone position, so that the contrast medium introduced into the oesophagus will be more likely to trickle anteriorly through a narrow fistula, under the influence of gravity, into the trachea. In this study non-ionic contrast media has been introduced via a catheter placed in the distal oesophagus. The catheter is slowly pulled back whilst injecting contrast. An H-type TOF has been opacified with contrast appearing in the trachea.

TOF may occur with or without oesophageal atresia. Oesophageal atresia most commonly occurs with a TOF (84%). In 6% TOF is present without oesophageal atresia and it is this type that exhibits the classic H-type fistula. Also oesophageal atresia occurs without a fistula in 9% seen as a gasless abdomen (Fig. 7b).

H-type fistulae without oesophageal atresia present later than pure oesophageal atresia. They may be difficult to image on conventional contrast studies, and an oesophagogram performed in the prone position with a feeding tube is the optimal way of demonstrating the fistula.

Oesophageal atresia may be associated with the presence of VATER or VACTERL anomalies where VATER/VACTERL stand for the following:

Vertebral anomalies
Anorectal atresia
Cardiovascular anomalies (ventricular septal defect (VSD), patent ductus arteriosus (PDA))
Tracheo-oesophageal fistula
Renal anomalies
Limb anomalies (radial ray hypoplasia, polydactyly)

In cases of oesophageal atresia with a TOF, immediate surgical repair is indicated. In oesophageal atresia without a TOF, if a long gap is present between the oesophageal ends surgery is usually deferred to allow growth of the oesophageal segments.

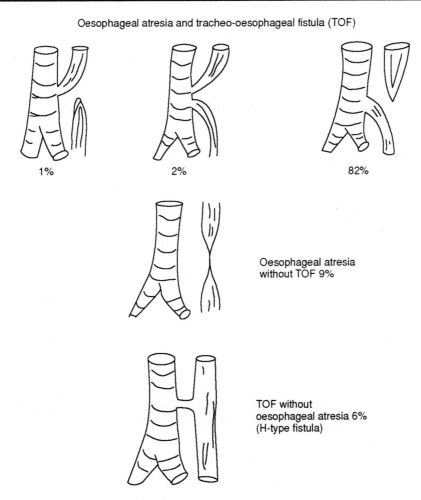

Oesophageal atresia and tracheo-oesophageal fistula (TOF)

1%   2%   82%

Oesophageal atresia
without TOF 9%

TOF without
oesophageal atresia 6%
(H-type fistula)

Fig. 7b   Congenital variants of oesophageal atresia and tracheo-oesophageal fistula.

Question 8

This 13-year-old boy was referred by his GP with a 2-month history of a painful limp. There was no history of trauma and he was systemically well. What does the anteroposterior (AP) pelvic radiograph (Fig. 8a) show? What are the potential complications?

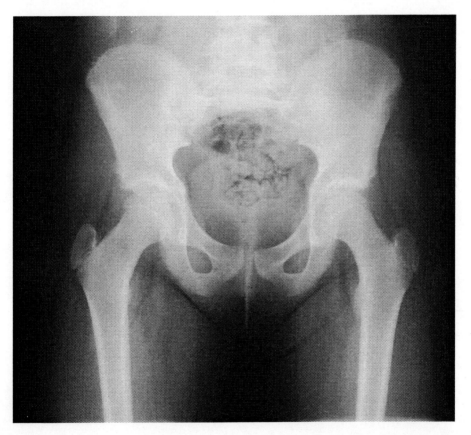

Fig. 8a

Answer 8: Left slipped capital femoral epiphysis (SCFE)

Potential complications: Avascular necrosis, chondrolysis, and premature osteoarthritis

Findings: There is posterior slip of the left capital femoral epiphysis. A straight line drawn along the lateral margin of the femoral neck should normally transect the superior aspect of the femoral epiphysis. On this radiograph (Fig. 8a) the left femoral epiphysis is not transected by this line. The frog-leg view (Fig. 8b) clearly shows the slip of the left capital femoral epiphysis.

Slipped capital femoral epiphysis (SCFE) is the most common adolescent hip disorder with boys affected 2–3 times more often than girls. SCFE is a Salter–Harris type 1 fracture of the proximal growth plate of the femur. It presents in males at ages 10–17 years and in girls at 8–15 years. Classically the patient is an overweight hypogonadal boy with delayed bone maturation. The condition is bilateral in 20–37% and therefore all patients should be closely followed up because about 25% develop a slip in the opposite hip within 18 months of the first slip.

Signs on pelvic radiograph:

- Posteromedial slip of the capital epiphysis with decreased epiphyseal height on the AP view;
- A line (Klein's line) drawn along the lateral femoral neck should intersect the capital epiphysis so that one-sixth of it lies lateral to the line on an AP radiograph;
- Irregularity and widening of the growth plate;
- Displacement of the femoral neck away from the acetabulum on the AP view. The medial third of the upper femoral neck should overlie the posterior aspect of the acetabulum;
- Inferomedial displacement of the femoral head relative to the metaphysis on frog-leg view (Fig 8b).

In 10% of cases no abnormality is detected on the AP film but the frog-leg view is usually diagnostic with inferomedial displacement of the epiphysis. The degree of slip may be graded as follows: grade I, less than one-third of the width of the neck; grade II, 33–50%; and grade III, > 50%.

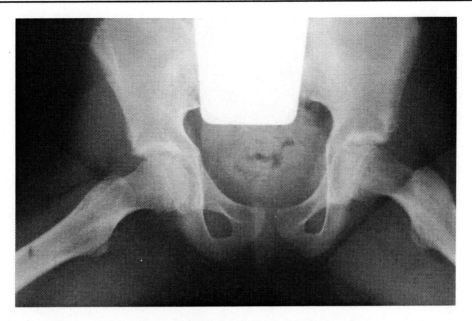

Fig. 8b Frog-leg view showing inferomedial slip of the left capital femoral epiphysis.

Question 9

This neonate (Fig. 9) developed respiratory distress. What is the diagnosis?

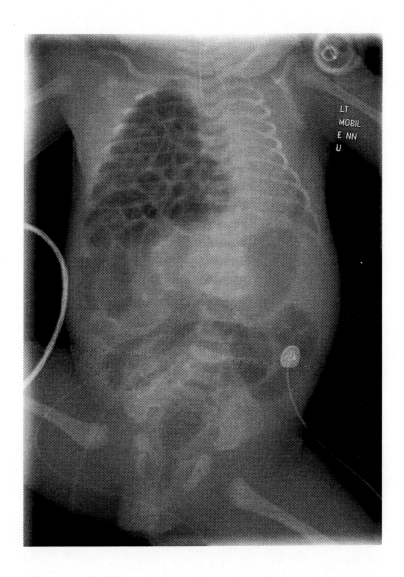

Fig. 9

Answer 9: Congenital diaphragmatic hernia

Findings: The right hemithorax is completely filled with bowel with resultant mediastinal shift to the left with compromise of left lung volume. The nasogastric tube could not be passed because of extrinsic oesophageal compression rather than an atresia and is curled up in the upper oesophagus.

The incidence of diaphragmatic hernia is 1 in 2500–3000 births. They are most commonly left-sided through the foramen of Bochdalek (85–90%). Diaphragmatic hernias usually present in the neonatal period with respiratory distress, although it is increasingly diagnosed antenatally. Associated anomalies (neural tube defects, malrotation, cardiovascular anomalies, trisomy 13 and 18, and intrauterine growth retardation) are present in 20% of live-births and 90% of stillbirths. The hernia usually contains bowel (small bowel 90%, stomach 60%, and colon 56%) but may contain spleen (54%), pancreas (24%), kidney, and liver. Poor prognostic signs include absence of contralateral aerated lung, a contralateral pneumothorax, and an intrathoracic stomach. Good prognostic features are greater than 50% aeration of the contralateral lung and presence of aerated lung ipsilateral to the hernia. Urgent surgical repair of the hernia is indicated.

Question 10

This 36-year-old man presented with haematuria and paroxysmal hypertension. He was on long-term follow-up for a hereditary condition. The figures show an axial contrast-enhanced CT section (Fig. 10a) and a coronal reformatted CT section (Fig. 10b) through the abdomen. What do the figures show? What is the underlying condition?

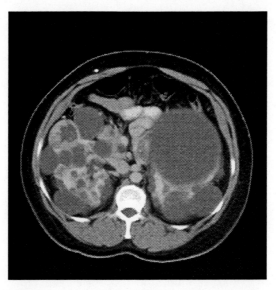

Fig. 10a

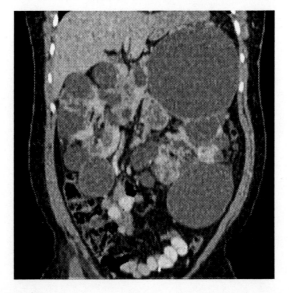

Fig. 10b

Answer 10: Von Hippel–Lindau (VHL) disease

Findings: Figure 10c (Fig. 10a reproduced) shows multiple cysts (arrows) throughout both kidneys. In the right kidney one of the cysts has a thickened enhancing wall consistent with a renal cell carcinoma (arrowheads). Note the ventriculo-peritoneal shunt running in the anterior abdominal wall (curved arrow) inserted for hydrocephalus secondary to the associated cerebellar haemangioblastomas. Figure 10d (Fig. 10b reproduced) shows a well-defined rim enhancing mass medial to the left kidney suspicious of a phaeochromocytoma (arrow).

VHL disease is an autosomal dominant condition due to a mutation of the VHL suppressor gene located at 3p 25:26. The age of onset is the second to third decade with an equal sex incidence.

Manifestations include:

- retinal angiomas (> 45%)
- cerebral haemangioblastomas (40%; the majority occur in the posterior fossa)
- renal cell carcinoma (20–45%)
- phaeochromocytoma (10–17%)
- pancreatic cystadenoma/cystadenocarcinoma

Cysts occur in mutiple organs including the liver, kidneys, pancreas, spleen, omentum, adrenals, lungs, and bone. The appearances of multiple visceral organ cysts may mimic adult polycystic renal disease. If a phaeochromocytoma is suspected on biochemical or radionuclide studies (I^{131} labelled metaiodobenzylguanidine (I^{131} MIBG) scan) patients must be adequately α and β receptor blocked prior to the administration of IV iodinated contrast agents to avoid a hypertensive crisis due to the sudden massive release of catecholamines.

Patients and their relatives are kept under close surveillance to identify and treat complications at a presymptomatic stage.

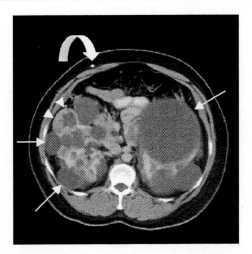

Fig. 10c   An axial contrast-enhanced CT section (Fig. 10a) showing multiple cysts throughout both kidneys (arrows). One of the cysts has a thickened enhancing wall consistent with a renal cell carcinoma (arrowheads). Note the ventriculo-peritoneal shunt (curved arrow) running in the anterior abdominal wall.

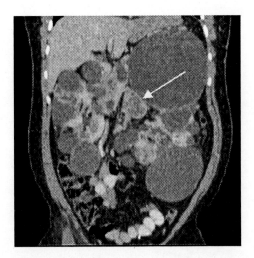

Fig. 10d   A coronal reformatted CT through the abdomen (Fig. 10b) showing a well defined rim-enhancing mass medial to the left kidney, suspicious of a phaeochromocytoma (arrow).

Question 11

This 45-year-old man presented to casualty after falling on his outstretched hand. AP and lateral hand radiographs are shown (Figs 11a and 11b, respectively). What is the diagnosis? What complications may occur?

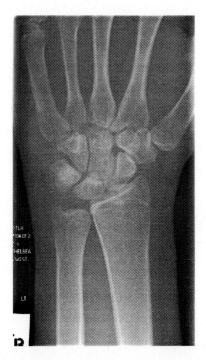

Fig. 11a

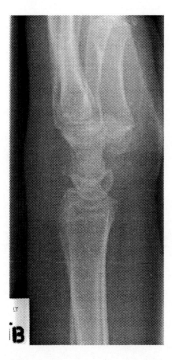

Fig. 11b

Answer 11: Triquetral fracture

Potential complications: Non-union, arthrosis, and carpal tunnel syndrome

Findings: The fracture is best seen on the lateral view as a bony fragment dorsal to the carpal bones. On the AP view there is a subtle cortical fracture of the triquetrum.

The triquetrum is the second most common carpal bone fractured after the scaphoid. The lateral view is the most useful in diagnosis as a fractured fragment can be seen dorsal to the wrist. In subtle injuries CT, MR, or radionuclide bone scans may be required. This case illustrates the importance of imaging trauma cases in two planes to avoid missing bony injuries.

Question 12

A 12-year-old boy presented to casualty with a painful ankle after falling off his bike. AP and lateral radiographs were performed (Figs 12a and 12b, respectively). What is the diagnosis? How would you classify this type of injury?

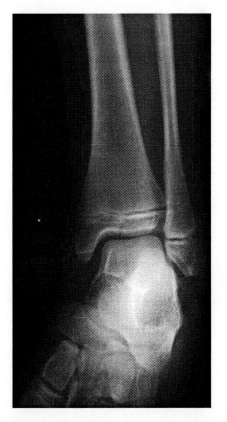

Fig. 12a

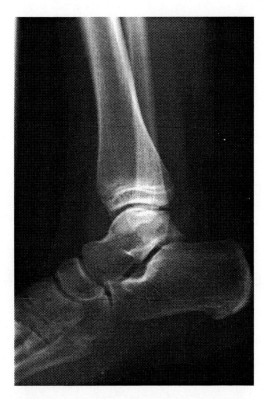

Fig. 12b

Answer 12: Salter–Harris Fracture type III

Findings: There is a vertical fracture through the distal tibial epiphysis (best seen on the AP view) consistent with a type III Salter–Harris fracture.

The epiphysis, epiphyseal plate, and metaphysis are involved in up to 15 % of fractures of the long bones in children. The epiphyseal plate is weaker than the adjacent ligaments and tendons and so is commonly involved in injuries. The complication of premature epiphyseal fusion may lead to angulation deformities or limb shortening. Such injuries are classified according to the Salter–Harris classification (Fig. 12c).

Salter–Harris classification:

Type I   Separation of the epiphysis with the fracture confined to the growth plate (6%). Examples include apophyseal avulsion and slipped capital femoral epiphysis. This has a good prognosis regardless of site.

Type II   Fracture through the growth plate extending through the metaphysis (75%). This type of fracture is usually seen at the distal radius and tibia. It has a good prognosis but may result in minimal shortening.

Type III   Fracture through the growth plate extending through the epiphysis (8%) and thus into the joint space. The prognosis is fair.

Type IV   Fracture extending from the articular surface of the epiphysis (i.e. involving the joint space) through the growth plate and metaphysis (10%). There is an increased likelihood of deformity and angulation.

Type V   Compression of the growth plate (1%). The prognosis is poor with growth impairment very common.

The prognosis is worse in the lower limb independent of Salter–Harris type.

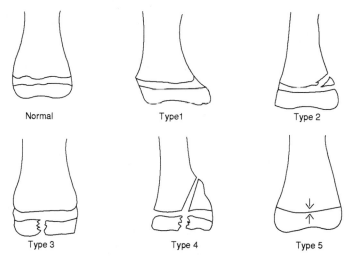

Fig. 12c   Salter–Harris classification of epiphyseal plate injuries.

Question 13

This 38-year-old man presented with acute right loin pain radiating to the groin. Urinalysis showed microscopic haematuria. An intravenous urogram (IVU) was performed. A 20 minute tomographic film from the IVU series is shown (Fig. 13). What is the diagnosis? What complication has occurred?

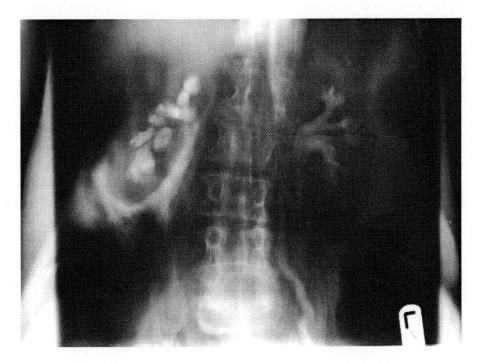

Fig. 13

Answer 13: Complete obstruction of the right kidney

Extravasation of contrast

Findings: Contrast medium tracks around the right kidney in the subcapsular and perinephric space. Contrast also tracks along the ureter. The right pelvicalyceal (PC) system is dilated indicating obstruction. The level of obstruction cannot be ascertained from this film but was subsequently shown to be in the distal ureter. The left upper renal tract is normal.

Spontaneous urinary extravasation occurs in approximately 4–8% of cases of acute ureteric obstruction. This is in the absence of any history of trauma or ureteric instrumentation. It is due to rupture of the collecting system at its weakest point, the calyceal fornix, where the calyx attaches to the papilla. The tears are usually due to a sudden increase in intrapelvic pressure. Extravasation has been shown to occur at pressures above 50 mmHg but the rate of pressure rise also appears to be important. In adults, the majority of cases are associated with ureteric calculi, whilst in children extravasation is mainly seen in posterior urethral valves and in pelvic–ureteric junction obstruction. Contrast enters the renal sinus, the space around the PC system, and may extend inferiorly to outline the ureter. Less commonly, contrast may track into the lymphatics, subcapsular region, perinephric space, or into the venous system (intravasation).

Usually extravasation is a benign process with spontaneous resolution unless the urine is infected. Most cases are due to a ureteric calculus that passes spontaneously. If the calculus fails to pass, nephrostomy or a ureteric stent may be required before a definitive procedure is performed to remove the stone. A urinoma may form in unrelieved obstruction. Management consists of drainage and correction of the obstruction.

Question 14

A 45-year-old man with known gallstones presented with sudden upper abdominal pain, nausea, and vomiting. A section from a contrast-enhanced abdominal CT is shown (Fig. 14). What is the diagnosis?

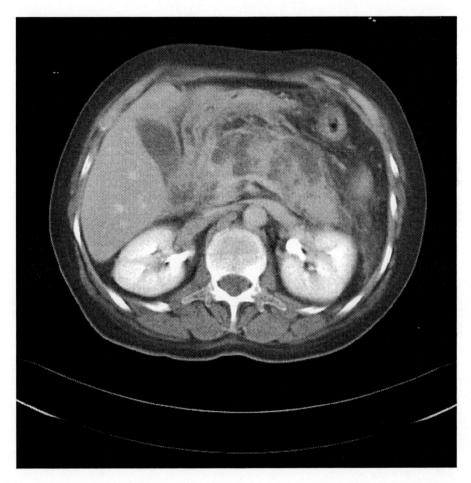

Fig. 14

Answer 14: Acute pancreatitis

Findings: The pancreas is oedematous with multiple low density areas in it consistent with necrosis. There is peripancreatic inflammatory change adjacent to the pancreatic tail.

Alcoholism and gallstones account for 90% of cases of acute pancreatitis. Other causes include hypercalcaemia, hyperlipidaemia, viral infections (mumps, coxsackie B), drugs (steroids), trauma, and congenital anomalies. The clinical presentation and course are variable, ranging from mild abdominal pain with nausea, vomiting, and abdominal distension to severe abdominal pain with multisystem failure and shock. Serum amylase levels are commonly analysed but are only elevated in 80–90% of cases and the degree of elevation does not correlate well with the severity of the inflammatory process.

Other radiological findings in acute pancreatitis are as follows.

- Chest X-ray (CXR) may show pleural effusion, basal atelectasis, diaphragmatic elevation, pulmonary air space opacity, or adult respiratory distress syndrome (ARDS).
- Abdominal X-ray (AXR) most commonly shows an abnormality of the intestinal gas pattern. This may be duodenal ileus (40%), a sentinel loop, or paucity of gas in the colon distal to the splenic flexure. Masses resulting from the pancreatitis may be identified through their displacement of intraabdominal structures.
- Ultrasound can demonstrate acute pancreatitis, but is less sensitive and specific than CT. Its main use is as a screening tool for biliary calculi or for follow-up of a known abnormality in patients with more severe disease.
- CT is the investigation of choice in patients with more severe disease or where a complication such as pseudocyst, infection, haemorrhage, pancreatic necrosis, or pseudoaneurysm is suspected.

The Glasgow (Imrie) scoring system is in widespread use and is a reliable predictor of severity. It measures eight parameters: age > 55 years; serum calcium (uncorrected) < 2 mmol/L; arterial pO_2 < 60 mmHg (8.0 kPa); blood glucose > 10 mmol/L; leucocytosis > 16×10^9/L; serum albumin < 32 g/L; serum urea > 16 mmol/L; and lactate dehydrogenase > 600 IU/L. One point is given for each positive parameter: a score of > 2 at 48 hours postonset predicts a severe outcome in 85% of cases. The Acute Physiology and Chronic Health Enquiry Score (APACHE II) measures multiple physiological parameters and a score of > 8 is an accurate predictor of a severe attack at admission.

Complications of acute pancreatitis include pseudocyst formation (10%), haemorrhage (3%), abscess formation (2–10%), biliary obstruction, ascites, thrombosis of the splenic and superior mesenteric veins, and pseudoaneurysm formation (10% of severe pancreatitis cases).

Question 15

This 76-year-old man presented with a history of change in bowel habit. What abnormality does the barium enema (Fig. 15) show?

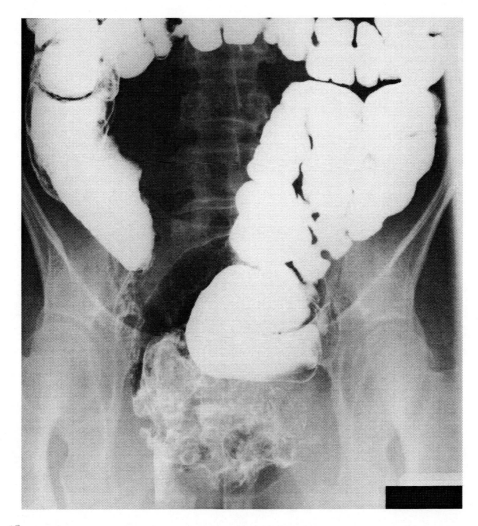

Fig. 15

Answer 15: Villous adenoma/polyp

Findings: There is a huge plaque-like lesion carpeting the rectosigmoid colon. The surface of the lesion is covered by innumerable mucosal fronds. Appearances are consistent with a villous adenoma.

Villous adenomas are most commonly located in the rectosigmoid colon (75%) and may completely encircle the colon. They are premalignant with the likelihood of malignant transformation dependent upon size: < 5 cm (9%); > 5 cm (55%); and > 10 cm (100%). Patients may present with rectal bleeding, excretion of copious mucus (may cause dehydration, hyponatraemia, and hypokalaemia), and tenesmus (sensation of incomplete evacuation).

Question 16

An 18-year-old lady presented with her third episode of abdominal pain and gastrointestinal bleeding. A gastroscopy was normal. Colonoscopy had revealed blood in the caecum but no source of bleeding was identified. A selective angiogram of the superior mesenteric artery (SMA) was performed (Fig. 16a). What does the angiogram show? What is the diagnosis?

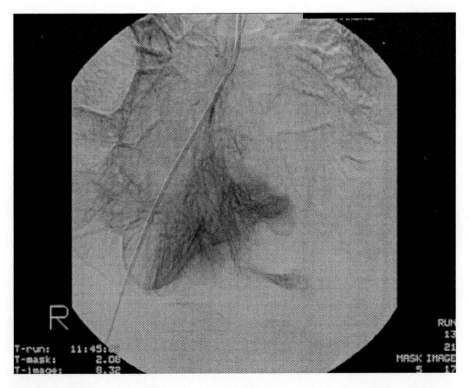

Fig. 16a

Answer 16: Meckel's diverticulum

Findings: The selective SMA angiogram shows a long vessel arising from one of the ileal branches extending caudally to supply an area of increased vascularity.

Catheterization of the above vessel shows it to be a persistent vitello-intestinal artery supplying a Meckel's diverticulum (arrow, Fig. 16b).

A Meckel's diverticulum is the vestigial remnant of the omphalomesenteric duct (vitelline duct). It is the most common gastrointestinal anomaly and occurs in 2–3% of the population. It usually presents in children under 2 years of age (M:F, 3:1). The diverticulum contains heterotopic tissue (ectopic gastric, pancreatic, or colonic mucosa). Ulceration, caused by secretion of hydrochloric acid and pepsin from the mucosal cells, results in gastrointestinal haemorrhage. A Meckel's diverticulum lies in the terminal six feet of the ileum in 94% and is usually approximately 2 inches long. A ^{99m}Tc-pertechnetate scan can also be used to detect a Meckel's diverticulum since the ectopic gastric mucosa takes up pertechnetate. Complications occur in 20% and include gastrointestinal haemorrhage, diverticulitis, bowel obstruction secondary to intussusception/fibrous bands, abdominal pain, and, rarely, malignant transformation.

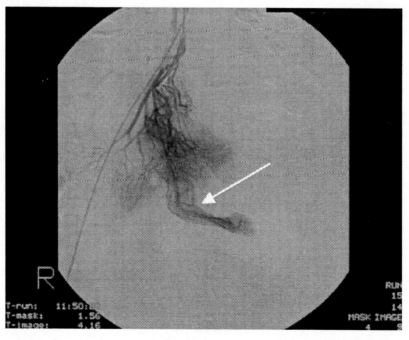

Fig. 16b   Angiogram showing a persistent vitello-intestinal artery supplying a Meckel's diverticulum (arrow).

Question 17

This 54-year-old lady presented with hypercalcaemia. What investigation (Fig. 17) has been performed? What is the diagnosis?

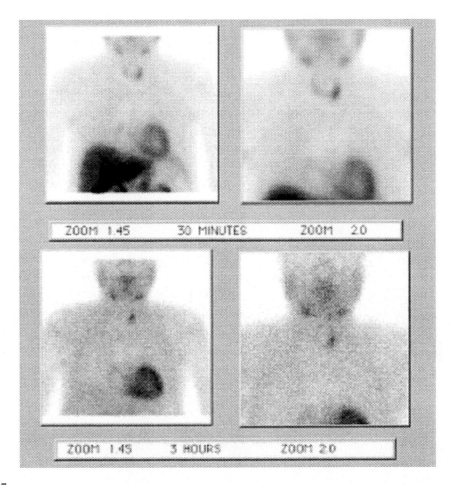

Fig. 17

Answer 17: ^{99m}Tc-sestamibi scan

Parathyroid adenoma (left inferior thyroid pole)

Findings: The anterior images of the thyroid have been obtained 30 minutes and 3 hours after an injection of ^{99m}Tc-sestamibi. The upper row images (30 minutes postinjection) demonstrate radiotracer accumulation in the thyroid and in the region of the inferior pole of the thyroid gland. On the 3 hour images (lower row) abnormal persistent activity in the region of the inferior pole of the thyroid is present while the rest of the thyroid activity has washed out. This is consistent with a parathyroid adenoma causing primary hyperparathyroidism. This was confirmed histologically.

Hyperparathyroidism is due to elevated parathormone (PTH) production. Primary, secondary, and tertiary hyperparathyroidism are recognized. Primary hyperparathyroidism is due to endogenous PTH hypersecretion caused by a solitary adenoma in 80% and by hyperplasia (usually of all four glands) in 10–15% and by carcinoma in 5%. Secondary hyperparathyroidism occurs in response to chronic hypocalcaemia (end-stage renal failure, malabsorption). Tertiary hyperparathyroidism occurs when one or more glands hypertrophy and become autonomous in secondary hyperparathyroidism.

The double phase ^{99m}Tc-sestamibi scan (early 10–30 minute and delayed 2–3 hour scan) is based on the more rapid tracer clearance from the normal thyroid compared with the abnormal parathyroid. Surgery is indicated if a parathyroid is identified and therefore reliable preoperative localization is essential. This technique is more accurate in identifying abnormal parathyroids than other radionuclide techniques, ultrasound, MR, and CT. It is also useful in detecting ectopic parathyroids, which occur in 10% of adenomas.

Question 18

This 7-year-old boy noticed a lump in the right groin. What does the coronal T1-weighted MR pelvis (Fig. 18a) show? What are the possible complications?

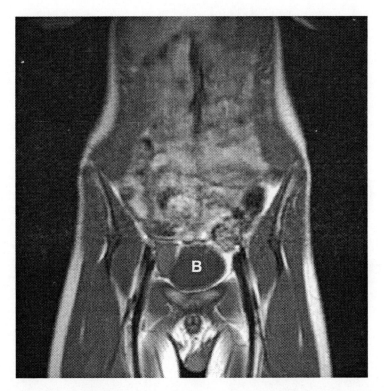

Fig. 18a Bladder (B) is indicated.

Answer 18: Right undescended testicle

Complications include an increased incidence of malignancy, sterility, and torsion.

Findings: The right undescended testicle is seen in the right inguinal canal (arrow, Fig. 18b). Note the presence of the normal left testicle in the scrotum.

The testes should normally be in the scrotum by 28–32 weeks gestation. However, approximately 86% of testes are normal in position at birth, with the vast majority of the remainder descending spontaneously by 1 year. Therefore the incidence of undescended testis is about 0.4% in men. Undescended testis may be divided into three groups: pseudocryptorchidism (70%; retractile testis due to spastic cremasteric muscle); cryptorchidism (20–29%; arrested descent of testis along its normal course); and ectopic testis (1%; deviation from the normal path). Ectopic testes pass through the inguinal canal and emerge from the superficial inguinal ring, thereafter following an abnormal course. In cryptorchidism the testis may be located in the high scrotum (50%), inguinal canal (20%), or abdomen (10%), whereas the ectopic testis may be sited in the abdominal wall, femoral triangle, perineum, or pubopenile region.

The risk of malignancy increases in an undescended testis, in a previously undescended testis, and in a normally descended testis with contralateral historical or current undescended testis. The risk of malignancy is increased by 30–50 times compared with the normal scrotal testis. Atrophic and intra-abdominal testes have an up to 200-fold increase in the incidence of malignancy. Tumours are most commonly seminomas and approximately 12% of testicular tumours arise in undescended testes.

The incidence of torsion is 10 times greater in cryptorchidism.

MR is the imaging modality of choice but other imaging strategies that may be employed to identify undescended testis include ultrasound (especially useful in testes sited in the inguinal canal), CT (maldescent is denoted by absence of the spermatic cord in the inguinal canal, although a testis < 1 cm cannot be reliably detected), and testicular venography. Laparoscopy is still the most reliable method of detecting an undescended testis.

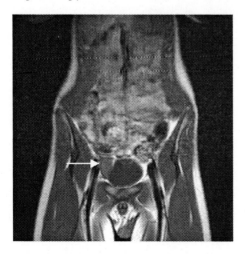

Fig. 18b   Coronal T1-weighted MR showing undescended testicle in the right inguinal canal (arrow). The normal left testicle is seen in the scrotum.

Question 19

This 76-year-old man underwent a recent cardiac catheterization procedure. A colour Doppler ultrasound examination (Fig. 19) was requested after he complained of groin pain. What is the diagnosis? What treatment options are available?

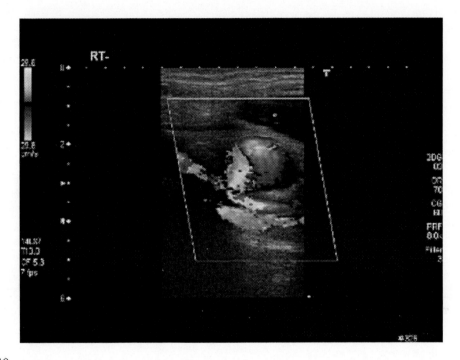

Fig. 19

Answer 19: Pseudoaneurysm of the right common femoral artery

Findings: There is a pseudoaneurysm arising from the anterior aspect of the right common femoral artery (CFA). Swirling turbulent flow is present in the pseudoaneurysm as shown by the mixed shaded pattern. It has a short neck and is therefore suitable for compression.

Treatment options:
1   Ultrasound (US)-guided compression;
2   US-guided percutaneous thrombin injection;
3   Surgical correction.

Local complications following a percutaneous catheterization include dissection, thrombosis, haematoma, pseudoaneurysm, and arteriovenous fistula. A pseudoaneurysm is a localized rupture of an artery contained by surrounding tissues. The wall of the pseudoaneurysm does not contain intima, media, and adventitia and this distinguishes it from a true aneurysm. Femoral artery pseudoaneurysms may be managed by US-guided compression to facilitate thrombosis. Criteria that predict success are a long and narrow track (< 5 mm) and a small collection. Longstanding injuries are more resistant to US-guided compression as are pseudoaneurysms that have short broad necks. US-guided percutaneous thrombin injection is an alternative if compression fails. US-guidance allows the needle tip to be sited in the centre of the sac, as far from the neck as possible, to avoid native artery thrombosis.

Question 20

This 26-year-old lady was involved in a road traffic accident and was taken to casualty complaining of back pain. Plain films and an MR of the thoracolumbar spine were performed. The lateral radiograph (Fig. 20a) and a sagittal T2-weighted MR of the thoracolumbar spine (Fig. 20b) are shown. What is the diagnosis? What associated injuries may be present?

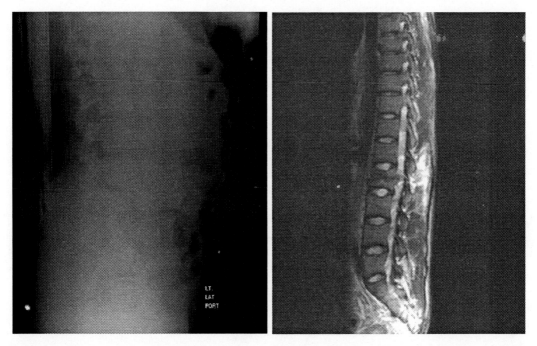

Fig. 20a   Fig. 20b

Answer 20: Chance fracture of L2

Findings: There is a wedge compression fracture of the vertebral body of L2. The sagittal MR confirms the vertebral body fracture and also shows that the fracture extends into the posterior elements. There is no dislocation of the fracture but there is some retropulsion of bony fragments into the spinal canal.

Potential associated injuries:
1 Vascular injury: thoracic/abdominal aortic injury; mesenteric vascular injuries;
2 Visceral injury: perforation of the jejunum and ileum > colon > duodenum. Abdominal visceral injury;
3 Soft tissue injury: tear of the rectus abdominis muscle; diaphragmatic injury;
4 Bone injury: rib, sternum and clavicle fractures.

The Chance fracture results from a shearing flexion-injury and is commonly seen in lap-type seatbelt injuries. It is characterized by a horizontal fracture of the spinous process, neural arch, and vertebral body. The L2/3 vertebrae are most commonly involved. Most Chance fractures are stable, but cord injury may occur, especially if there is dislocation. The radiographic findings of a Chance fracture may be subtle. Pedicles and spinous processes should be inspected for cortical fractures. Extension through the vertebral body may result in irregularity of the superior or inferior endplates. Widening of the spinous processes with anterior angulation of the vertebral body is suspicious of a Chance fracture. These fractures may be missed on CT because the fracture runs parallel to the horizontal scan axis. Thus fractures are best depicted by MR. Intra-abdominal injuries occur in approximately 40% of cases with a higher incidence of intestinal injuries in children.

Question 21

This 64-year-old patient presented acutely with a urinary tract infection (UTI). What complication of a UTI does this intravenous urogram (Fig. 21) show?

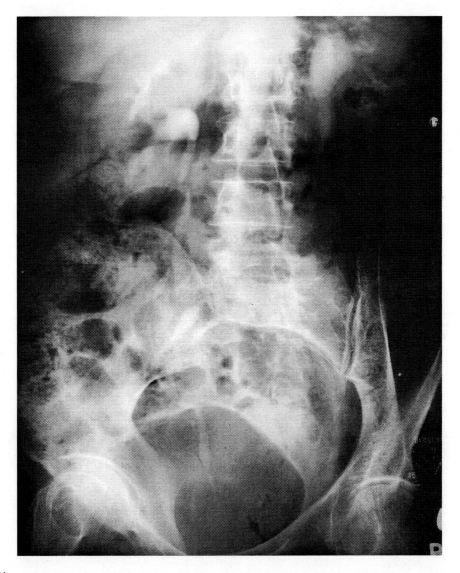

Fig. 21

Answer 21: Emphysematous cystitis

Findings: The bladder is full of gas. Both pelvicalyceal systems are normal with prompt and symmetrical excretion of contrast. The whole length of the right ureter is seen, compatible with hold-up at the right vesicoureteric junction presumably secondary to oedema.

Emphysematous cystitis is due to infection by gas-forming organisms (usually *E. coli*) and the gas is usually localized to the bladder submucosa. The example depicted is a particularly florid case with the bladder full of gas. It is more common in females and predisposing conditions include diabetes mellitus, immunocompromised state, bladder outflow obstruction, and neurogenic bladder. The condition is analogous to emphysematous pyelonephritis but has a lower morbidity/mortality. Symptoms include dysuria, frequency, and pneumaturia. Treatment consists of antibiotics, control of diabetes, and relief of obstruction if present. The plain film is often diagnostic with linear streaks of submucosal gas, but CT demonstrates the thickened bladder wall and intramural gas. Ultrasound also depicts the thickened bladder wall and the mural gas is seen as echogenic foci with acoustic shadowing. Gas in the bladder lumen may have multiple causes (e.g. instrumentation, fistula formation, trauma, and infection), but gas in the bladder wall is pathognomonic of infection with a gas-forming organism.

Question 22

This 44-year-old postman complained of pain on walking. What does this plain radiograph (Fig. 22a) show?

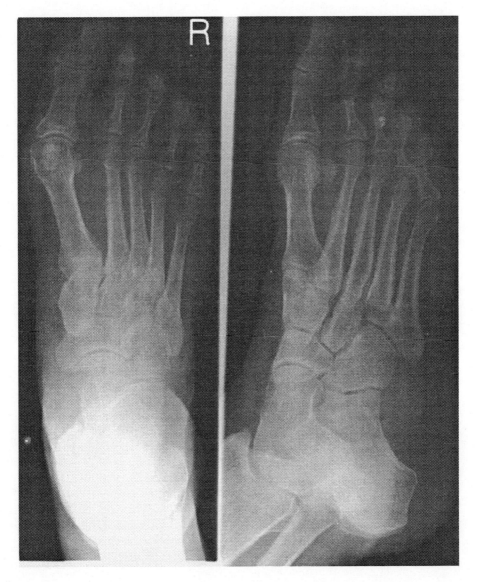

Fig. 22a

Answer 22: Stress fracture of the shaft of the second metatarsal

Findings: There is a subtle periosteal reaction along the midshaft of the second metatarsal with no fracture visible, consistent with a stress (march) fracture. On the follow-up radiograph 6 weeks later the fracture is obvious (Fig. 22b).

Stress fractures may be divided into fatigue fractures, where an abnormal stress is applied to a bone with normal mineralization, or insufficiency fractures, in which normal physiological stress results in fracture of a bone with deficient mineralization. Examples of fatigue fractures include the following.

1 Metatarsal as in the case illustrated: seen in marching, ballet, and prolonged standing;
2 Navicular: marching, ballet;
3 Calcaneus: jumping, parachuting;
4 Tibial shaft: ballet, jogging;
5 Fibula: jogging, jumping, parachuting;
6 Femoral neck/shaft: ballet, marching, jogging;
7 Spondylolysis: pars interarticularis in ballet, weight-lifting;
8 Hook of hamate: golfers and racquet sports;
9 Clay shoveller's fracture of the spinous process of the lower cervical/upper thoracic spine;
10 Coracoid process of the scapula in trap shooting;
11 Distal humeral shaft/coronoid process of the ulna in ball throwing sports.

In the early stage of the fracture diagnosis is very difficult. Bone scan and MR allow much earlier diagnosis if the condition is suspected clinically.

Insufficiency fractures occur in osteoporosis, osteomalacia, Paget's disease, metabolic bone diseases such as hyperparathyroidism, renal osteodystrophy, and radiation therapy. Fractures most commonly occur in the lower limb, sacrum, ilium, and pubic bone.

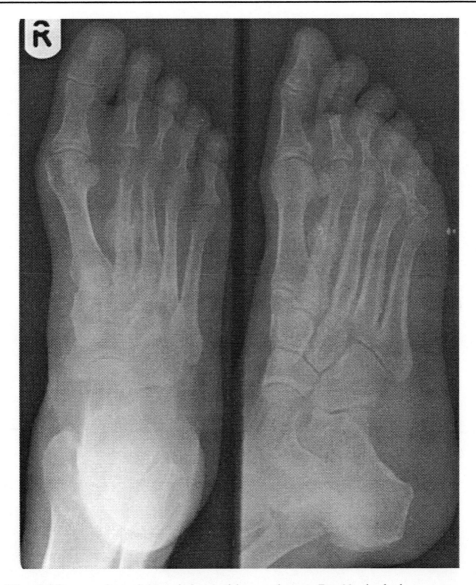

Fig. 22b   A follow-up radiograph (6 weeks later) of the case shown in Fig. 22a clearly shows a stress fracture of the shaft of the second metatarsal.

Question 23

This neonate presented with acute bilious vomiting. What does the barium meal (Fig. 23) show?

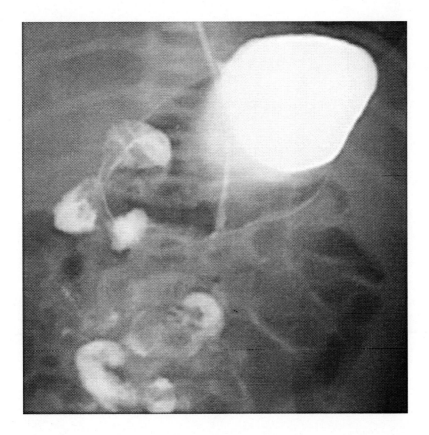

Fig. 23

Answer 23: Malrotation with volvulus

Findings: The barium meal shows a proximal small bowel obstruction with a spiral/corkscrew configuration of the duodenum and jejunum. The duodeno-jejunal (DJ) flexure is abnormally positioned, lying in the midline, rather than to the left of the midline at the level of the gastric antrum.

Malrotation complicated by volvulus usually presents in the first month of life and is a paediatric emergency because of the risk of bowel ischaemia and infarction. Malrotation covers a wide spectrum of anomalies of intestinal rotation and fixation. The DJ flexure should lie to the left of the midline at the level of the gastric antrum. If the ligament of Trietz and caecum are poorly fixed the short mesentery predisposes to midgut volvulus. As well as the classic features on barium meal above, ultrasound or CT may show the 'whirlpool sign' of the superior mesenteric vein (SMV) wrapped around the SMA. A Ladd operation is performed to reduce the volvulus, resect infarcted bowel, and lyse dense peritoneal Ladd's bands.

Malrotation results from arrest of the normal embryonic gut rotation and fixation. These patients have a narrow mesenteric attachment. Normally, the primitive bowel rotates 270 degrees counterclockwise. By definition, rotation of < 90 degrees is 'non-rotation' (0.2% of adults) and rotation of 90–270 degrees is 'malrotation'. With non-rotation, the small bowel lies on the right side of the abdomen and the colon on the left. CT or ultrasound shows an abnormal orientation of the superior mesenteric artery and vein, with the vein lying to the left of the artery (80%), i.e. the opposite of their normal juxtaposition where the artery lies to the left of the vein.

Question 24

This 6-year-old boy presented with difficulty in walking. A pelvic radiograph (Fig. 24) is shown. What is the diagnosis?

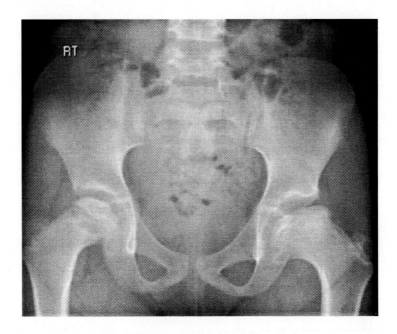

Fig. 24

Answer 24: Perthe's disease

Findings: There is sclerosis and partial collapse of both femoral capital epiphyses, more marked on the left. There is widening of the joint space bilaterally due to effusions.

Perthe's disease is due to idiopathic avascular necrosis of the femoral head and occurs between the ages of 4 and 10 years. It is more common in males and is bilateral in 10%. The natural history of the disease may be divided into two phases: evolution and healing. The bone usually returns to normal but there may be considerable deformation of the femoral head and neck.

Plain film radiographic signs include the following:

- The earliest sign is widening of the joint space with a small capital femoral epiphysis;
- Subcortical lucency or fissuring of the epiphysis;
- Later progressive flattening, fragmentation, and sclerosis of the femoral heads occur;
- Late features include remodelling of the femoral head and neck.

Bone scintigraphy is more sensitive than plain films in the detection of early cases when a photopenic defect is present corresponding to the avascular area. MR is also very sensitive in the early stages of the disease. Most patients respond well to conservative treatment. However, premature osteoarthritis is a recognized complication in early adulthood.

Question 25

This 84-year-old lady presented with a change in bowel habit. An image from a barium enema is shown (Fig. 25). What is the diagnosis? What are the possible causes?

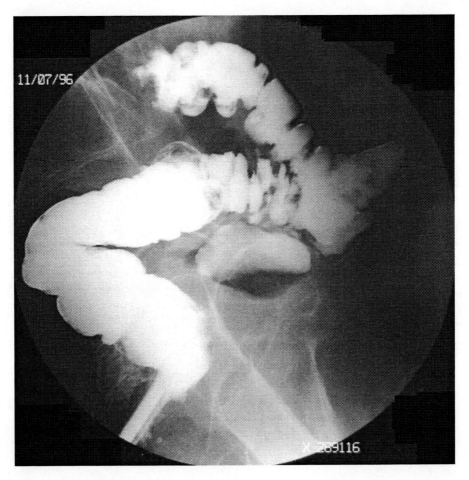

Fig. 25

Answer 25: Colovesical fistula due to sigmoid diverticulitis

Findings: There is severe sigmoid diverticular disease resulting in a long narrow irregular segment. Barium is seen in the bladder, with an air fluid level, consistent with a colovesical fistula.

Causes of colonic fistulae:

- inflammatory conditions, e.g. diverticulitis, Crohn's disease;
- neoplastic, e.g. carcinoma of the colon or cervix;
- infection, e.g. TB, abscesses;
- instrumentation;
- trauma;
- radiotherapy.

Patients with colovesical fistulae present with pneumaturia and with recurrent urinary tract infections due to bowel organisms. The fistula may be imaged by barium enema or a cystogram. Cystoscopy may reveal faecal material and/or bubbles entering the bladder from the fistula. Management depends on the cause but surgical resection of the diverticular disease is usually sufficient. The bladder defect is usually indiscernible and can be managed with a urinary catheter postoperatively.

Question 26

This film (Fig. 26) was part of a screening mammogram performed on a 65-year-old lady. What is the diagnosis? Should she be referred for biopsy?

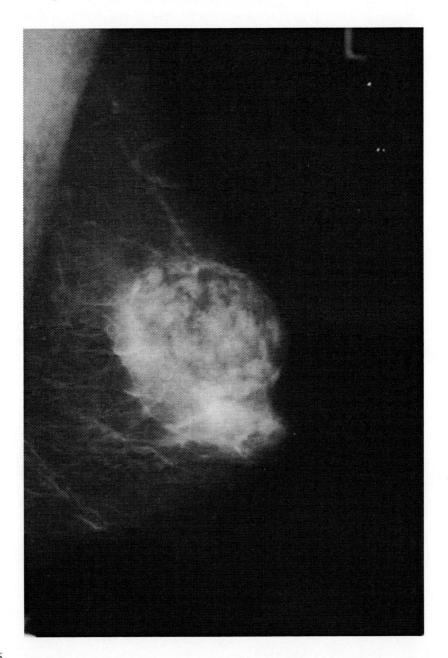

Fig. 26

Answer 26: Fibroadenolipoma (hamartoma)

Biopsy is unnecessary as hamartomas are benign.

Findings: There is an encapsulated, well circumscribed mass composed of mixed radiolucent and radiodense areas. There is no distortion of the adjacent tissue. Appearances are pathognomonic of a hamartoma. The appearances have been likened to a 'slice of sausage'.

Fibroadenolipomas (hamartomas) are uncommon, benign breast tumours containing glandular, fat, and fibrous tissue in varying proportions. They are surrounded by a thin capsule of connective tissue. Their size may vary from millimetres to lesions that occupy most of the breast. When palpable, hamartomas are mobile and smooth. Ultrasound is rarely helpful in the evaluation of a hamartoma since mammographic appearances are characteristic.

Question 27

This neonate was noted to have bilateral hydronephrosis on antenatal ultrasound. Postnatally, a micturating cystourethrogram (MUCG; Fig. 27a) was performed. What is the diagnosis?

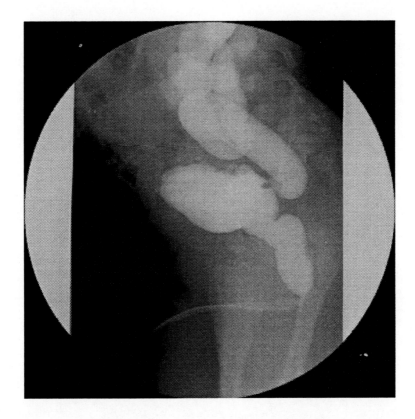

Fig. 27a

Answer 27: Posterior urethral valves

Findings: Figure 27b (Fig. 27a reproduced) shows dilatation of the posterior urethra (arrows) with posterior urethral valves present (arrowhead). The bladder is thick-walled and trabeculated secondary to bladder outlet obstruction. The anterior urethra is normal. Ureteric reflux is present.

Posterior urethral valves are thickened mucosal folds distal to the verumontanum and are the most common cause of bilateral hydronephrosis in a male infant. Posterior urethral valves only occur in males and usually present in the neonatal period (34%) or first year (32%). Presenting features include obstructive symptoms (straining, hesitancy, dribbling), urinary tract infection, and failure to thrive. They may also present with pulmonary hypoplasia and cystic renal dysplasia. Posterior urethral valves are now increasingly suspected on antenatal ultrasound with maternal oligohydramnios, dilated upper renal tracts, and a thick-walled bladder.

Vesicoureteric reflux (more common on the left) may lead to hydronephrosis and renal dysplastic changes. Calyceal leak may result in urinoma and ascites. The management is cystoscopic valve resection/ablation.

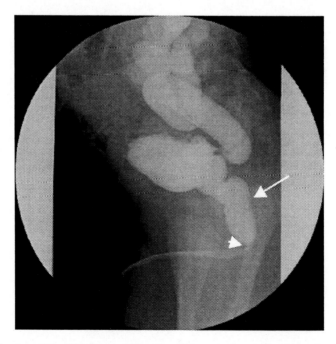

Fig. 27b   Reproduction of Fig. 27a showing dilatation of the posterior urethra (arrow) with posterior urethral valves present (arrowhead).

Question 28

This 25-year-old man presented with a painless swelling in the left testicle. What two abnormalities does this transverse testicular ultrasound (Fig. 28) show?

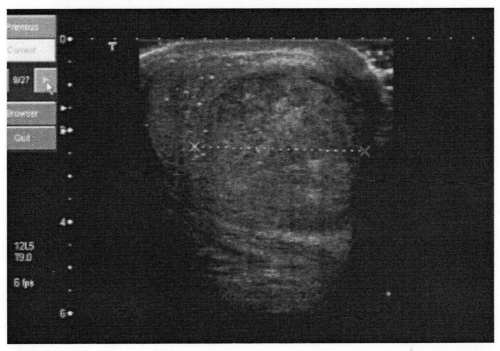

Fig. 28

Answer 28: *Testicular microlithiasis and a tumour (between callipers)*

Findings: There is a mass of heterogeneous echotexture in the testis consistent with a tumour. Testicular microlithiasis is also present (seen as 'starry night' appearance in the top left of the testicle).

Testicular microlithiasis (TM) is due to formation of calcium deposits from degenerating cells in the seminiferous tubules. The ultrasound appearances are of tiny (< 2 mm) echogenic foci that do not produce acoustic shadowing. TM is associated with Klinefelter's syndrome, cryptorchidism, subfertility, and Down syndrome. TM is also associated with malignant tumours, seminomas being the most frequently seen. *In situ* premalignant intratubular germ cell neoplasia is also more common. If TM is discovered incidentally, ultrasound follow-up is necessary. A consensus on the frequency and duration of this follow-up has not been reached.

Question 29

This 27-year-old male intravenous drug addict presented with a 2 month history of pain in the left thigh. The plain radiograph (Fig. 29a) and an axial T2-weighted MR (Fig. 29b) of the left thigh are shown. What is the diagnosis?

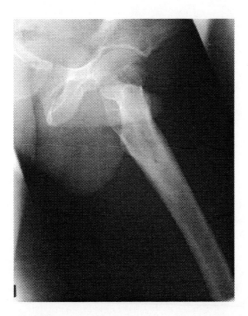

Fig. 29a

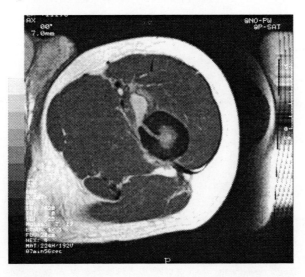

Fig. 29b

Answer 29: Chronic osteomyelitis with a draining sinus

Findings: The plain radiograph shows an ill-defined area of sclerosis in the proximal femur with a periosteal reaction and a small round cortical lucency (sinus). The MR (Fig. 29c) shows an area of high signal in the medulla consistent with bone marrow oedema. There is a sinus (arrow Fig. 29c) leading to a small collection in the anterior muscular compartment (open arrow, Fig. 29c).

Osteomyelitis may be acute, subacute, or chronic. Osteomyelitis affects mainly the epiphysis in infants and adults and the metaphysis in children. The route of dissemination may be haematogenous; direct spread from adjacent structures, e.g. septic arthritis; penetrating injury; or surgery. The most common organism is *Staphylococcus aureus* in immunocompetent adults with *Pseudomonas*, *Klebsiella*, and *Enterobacteriae* commonly seen in drug addicts.

In acute osteomyelitis plain radiographs are often normal for as long as 10 days. MR is very sensitive in the detection of early osteomyelitis. The MR features of acute osteomyelitis include low signal on T1-weighted sequences in the normally high signal marrow and high signal on T2-weighted and inversion-recovery sequences consistent with bone marrow oedema. Triple phase bone scintigraphy is sensitive but not specific. A negative scan virtually excludes the diagnosis. White cell scans are more specific than bone scintigraphy.

In chronic osteomyelitis, prominent cortical thickening and periosteal reaction are seen with a mixed pattern of osteosclerosis and osteolysis. A draining sinus and sequestrum (detached necrotic cortical bone) may be present.

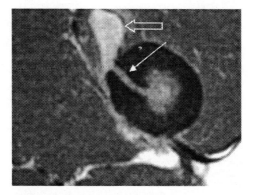

Fig. 29c   The axial T2-weighted MR shows an area of high signal in the medulla consistent with bone marrow oedema. There is a sinus (arrow) leading to a small collection in the anterior muscular compartment (open arrow).

Question 30

This 57-year-old lady gave a 6-month history of abdominal pain, diarrhoea, and flushing. A contrast-enhanced CT image of the abdomen (Fig. 30a) is shown. What are the abnormal findings? What is the diagnosis?

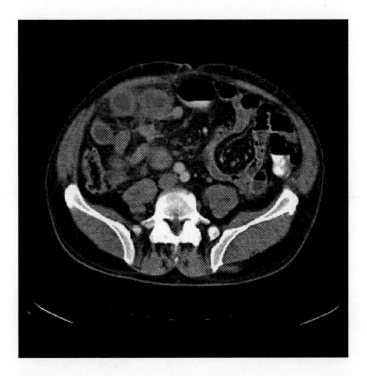

Fig. 30a

Answer 30: Carcinoid

Findings: There are thickened small bowel loops (chevrons). There is also a mass (arrow) in the mesentery of the small bowel with stranding (arrowheads) and distortion of the surrounding fat consistent with an associated fibrotic desmoplastic reaction (Fig. 30b).

Given the history of flushing and diarrhoea, carcinoid is the most likely diagnosis. Carcinoid is a tumour of the APUD (amine precursor uptake and decarboxylation) system. It is the most common tumour of the small bowel and appendix. One-third occur in the small bowel (30–45% in the appendix), more commonly in ileum than jejunum, one-third have metastases, one-third are multifocal, and one-third have a second malignancy. Carcinoid syndrome is caused by secretion of excess serotonin (5-hydroxytryptamine), which is usually converted to 5-hydroxyindoleacetic acid (5-HIAA) in the liver. When this filter mechanism is bypassed in the presence of liver metastases or lung involvement, carcinoid syndrome occurs with diarrhoea, flushing, asthma, hypotension, nausea and vomiting, and right-sided heart failure. In both metaiodobenzylguanidine (I-123 MIBG) and octreotide scintigraphy, the radiopharmaceuticals are taken up by carcinoid tumours and this technique is useful in monitoring disease.

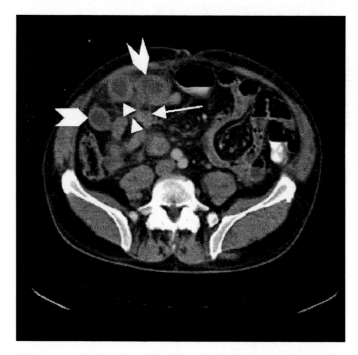

Fig. 30b   Contrast-enhanced CT image of the abdomen showing thickened small bowel loop (chevrons) in the right iliac fossa. There is also a mass (arrow) in the mesentery of the small bowel with stranding (arrowheads) and distortion of the surrounding fat consistent with an associated fibrotic desmoplastic reaction.

Question 31

What does this intravenous urogram (Fig. 31) show?

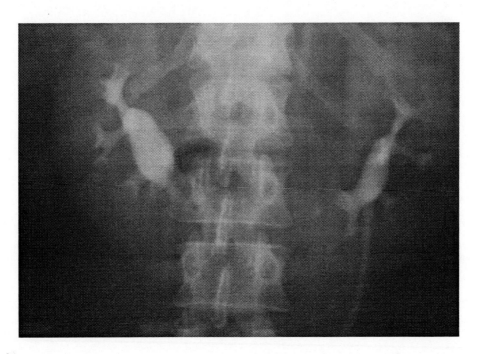

Fig. 31

Answer 31: Horseshoe kidney

Findings: The inferior renal poles are united by a bridge of tissue that lies below the inferior mesenteric artery which impedes the normal embryological ascent. Therefore the kidneys are lower than normal in the abdomen. The lower calyces on each side point medially instead of laterally.

Horseshoe kidneys have an incidence of 0.2–1% and a male predominance (male:female 2:1). It is the most common renal fusion anomaly. Fusion occurs at the lower poles in 90% by a parenchymal (most common) or fibrous isthmus. The condition is associated with cardiovascular and skeletal anomalies, anorectal malformation, genitourinary anomalies (hypospadias, undescended testis, bicornuate uterus, and ureteric duplication), trisomy 18, and Turner's syndrome.

The pelviureteric junction faces anteriorly instead of medially and so the ureter has to run anteriorly to cross the joining bridge between the kidneys. This impairs urinary drainage and the resultant urinary stasis leads to an increased incidence of obstruction, infection, and calculi. Horseshoe kidneys also have an increased incidence of vesicoureteric reflux, Wilms' tumour, and susceptibility to trauma, the latter because the kidneys are more superficial and are anterior to the lumbar spine.

Question 32

This 62-year-old lady underwent mammography (Fig. 32a) as part of a breast screening programme. What is the diagnosis?

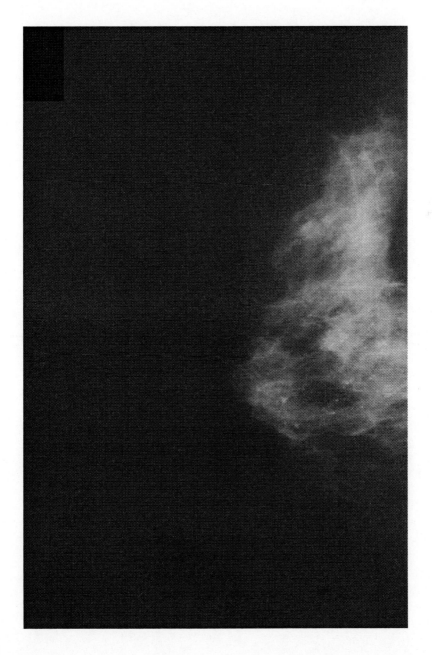

Fig. 32a

Answer 32: *Ductal carcinoma* in situ *(DCIS)*

Findings: There is pleomorphic microcalcification in the right breast. The calcifications vary in size and density and have irregular linear branching patterns. They are aligned in the ductal system. There is no discrete mass. DCIS was confirmed on biopsy.

Breast cancer may have a spectrum of mammographic appearances. DCIS consists of two types.

1   Comedo type (60% of DCIS) is characterized histologically by central necrosis in the involved ducts. Comedo carcinoma *in situ* may be present alone or with invasive carcinoma. The high-grade comedo-type DCIS has a higher incidence of recurrence then the non-comedo-type.
2   Non-comedo type (40% of all DCIS) is of lower grade than the comedo type.

Of cases of DCIS, 20–50% will develop invasive carcinoma in 10 years. If more than 25% of the breast is involved, mastectomy may be necessary. Mastectomy has a cure rate of almost 100%.

In contrast, an invasive ductal carcinoma is shown opposite (Fig. 32b) as a spiculated mass with adjacent skin thickening (peau d'orange) and tethering.

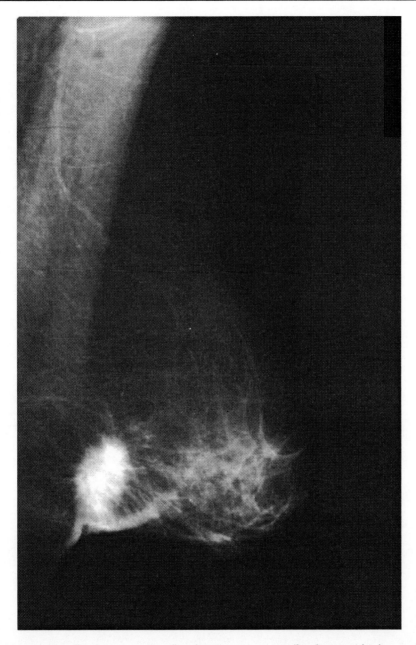

Fig. 32b   Mammogram showing an invasive ductal carcinoma as a spiculated mass with adjacent skin thickening and tethering.

Question 33

This 36-year-old man presented acutely with a haematemesis. He declined an endoscopy. A barium meal was performed (Fig. 33a). Describe the findings? What is the diagnosis? What complications are associated with this lesion?

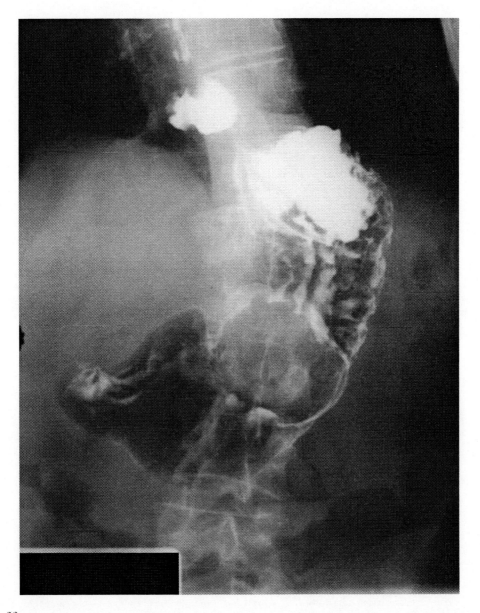

Fig. 33a

Answer 33: Gastric gastrointestinal stromal tumour (GIST; formerly known as leiomyma)

Findings: There is a well-defined smooth filling defect that does not distort the adjacent gastric rugae or mucosal pattern.

Asszociated complications are:

- haemorrhage (may be massive);
- obstruction (may cause intussusception);
- perforation/fistulation;
- malignant change.

GIST is the most common kind of mesenchymal neoplasm of the alimentary tract, 60–70% arise in the stomach. Gastric GIST is the second most common benign tumour of the stomach after polyps. These tumours are submucosal (60%), exophytic subserosal (35%), or are dumbbell-shaped (extra and intramural) in 5%. Classically, gastric GISTs are ovoid with a smooth margin, and are approximately 4 cm in size and have central ulceration ('bull's eye' sign) in 50%. CT (Fig. 33b) is useful preoperatively as these tumours exhibit the 'iceberg phenomenon' with a large extraluminal component that would be unsuspected on a barium meal study. Calcification is present in 4%. The prediction of malignancy of GIST is difficult; the only reliable indications being the presence of local invasion or distant metastases at the time of diagnosis.

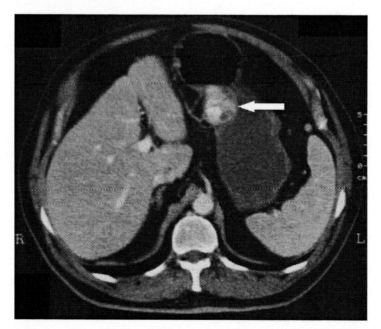

Fig. 33b   CT section through the upper abdomen showing the intraluminal portion of a partially calcified gastric gastrointestinal stromal tumour (GIST) (arrow). The extraluminal component (not shown) extended to lie anterior to the pancreas.

Question 34

This 76-year-old lady presented with a change in bowel habit. What abnormality is demonstrated on the barium enema (Fig. 34)?

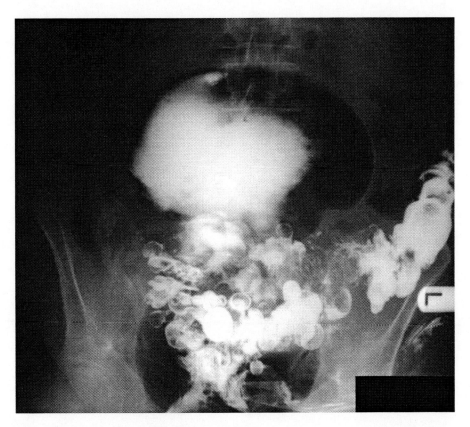

Fig. 34

Answer 34: A giant sigmoid diverticulum

Findings: There is a large gas/barium-containing diverticulum communicating with a segment of sigmoid diverticular disease. The differential diagnosis would be an abscess.

Giant sigmoid diverticulae have the same aetiology as all colonic diverticulae but are thought to enlarge markedly secondary to a ball-valve phenomenon. Complications that may occur are:

- infection;
- perforation;
- fistulation;
- haemorrhage.

Question 35

This 55-year-old lady had undergone lumpectomy for a previous carcinoma of the right breast. The follow-up mammogram (mediolateral view) is shown (Fig. 35a). What abnormality is present?

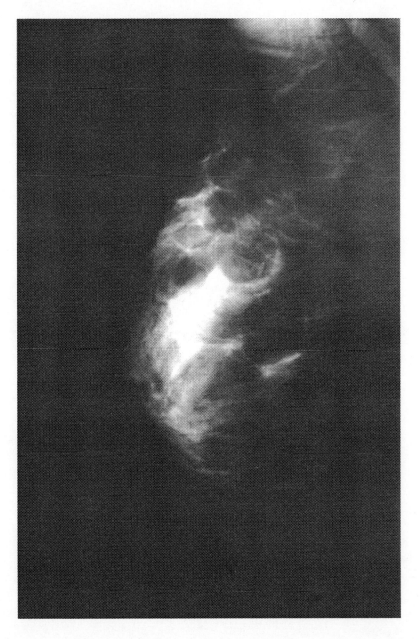

Fig. 35a

Answer 35: Oil cyst (fat necrosis secondary to surgery)

Findings: There is a well defined, lucent, oval lesion (arrow, Fig. 35b) with a smooth wall. This has the appearance of an oil cyst. A small opacity that represents postsurgical change is seen inferior to the oil cyst. This is no evidence of tumour recurrence.

Fat necrosis of the breast is a benign condition characterized by nonsuppurative inflammatory response to surgery, trauma, biopsy, and radiotherapy. Patients are usually asymptomatic, but may present with a palpable mass (painful or painless) with erythema, skin thickening, and retraction.

The mammographic appearances of fat necrosis have a wide spectrum, ranging from a well-defined oil cyst to spiculated masses that mimic carcinoma. The calcification ranges from microcalcification (pleomorphic) to large, coarse, plaque-like or eggshell calcification that has a more benign appearance. Mammographic follow-up and sometimes biopsy may be necessary in difficult cases.

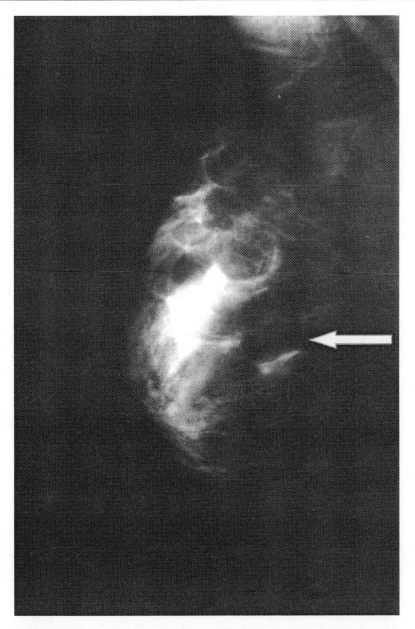

Fig. 35b   Mammogram showing a well-defined lucent, oval lesion with a smooth wall, which has the appearance of an oil cyst (arrow).

Question 36

This 26-year-old lady presented with vague pelvic pain that had been present for 8 months. What does the contrast-enhanced pelvic CT section (Fig. 36a) show?

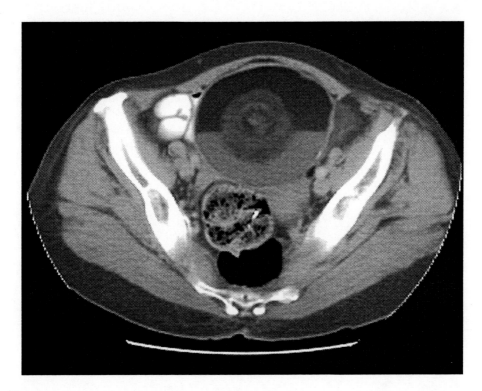

Fig. 36a

Answer 36: Ovarian dermoid

Findings: There is a spherical, encapsulated mass lying anteriorly in the pelvis with a fat-fluid level (arrows) and a soft tissue Rokitansky nodule (N) floating in the lesion (Fig. 36b). The appearances are pathognomonic of an ovarian dermoid.

A dermoid cyst, or mature cystic teratoma, is the most common ovarian neoplasm. It is a benign tumour composed of tissues arising from all three germ cell layers. They are bilateral in 10–25%. They may present with an abdominal mass or abdominal pain due to torsion, rupture, or haemorrhage. The presence of a fat-fluid level or calcification (teeth or bone) is diagnostic. A Rokitansky nodule (dermoid plug) consisting of hair, fat, and calcium is seen in 81% on CT. Dermoids, although benign, are always removed because of their propensity to undergo torsion and malignant change (usually squamous cell carcinoma in the elderly) in 1–3%.

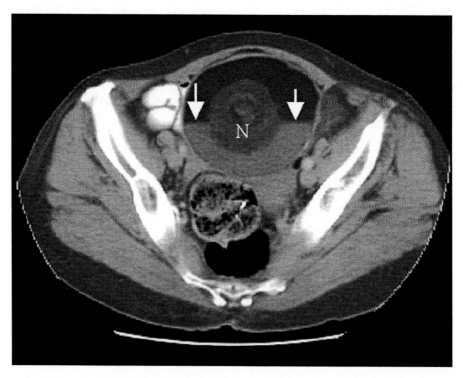

Fig. 36b   Contrast-enhanced pelvic CT section showing a spherical encapsulated mass lying anteriorly in the pelvis with a fat-fluid level (arrows) and a soft tissue Rokitansky nodule (N) floating in the lesion.

Question 37

This examination (Fig. 37a) was performed as part of routine preoperative assessment prior to coronary artery bypass surgery. What is the examination? What does the image show?

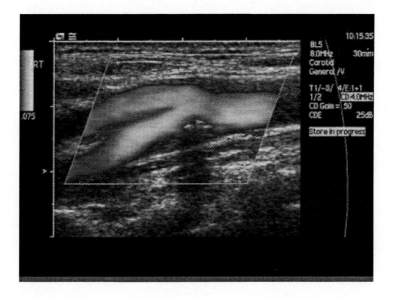

Fig. 37a

Answer 37: Proximal internal carotid artery stenosis

The image is from a carotid Doppler ultrasound.

Findings: The image (Fig. 37b) shows a plaque in the carotid bulb, extending into the origin of the internal carotid artery, resulting in a stenosis. The common carotid artery (CCA), internal carotid artery (ICA), and external carotid artery (ECA) are indicated.

Stroke is the third most common cause of death in the UK. One-third of acute strokes are fatal. High-grade ICA stenosis (> 70%) is associated with an increase in the incidence of stroke, transient ischaemic attack (TIA), and cerebral emboli. In 1991 the North American Symptomatic Carotid Endarterectomy Trial (NASCET) and the European Carotid Surgery Trial (ECST) showed that, in symptomatic patients with a stenosis of greater than 70%, carotid endarterectomy produced a significant reduction in stroke compared with conservative therapy. The ECST trial showed that, during the follow-up period, the percentage of subjects having ischaemic symptoms lasting more than 7 days was 16.8% for those on medical management, compared with 2.8% if surgery was performed. With intermediate degrees of stenoses (30–69%), the ESCT data showed no advantage of surgery. In asymptomatic patients with stenoses of greater than 60%, the Asymptomatic Carotid Atherosclerosis Study (ACAS) showed that surgery reduced the risk of subsequent stroke by 5% provided that the centre had a perioperative mortality of less than 3%. However, more recent meta-analyses have shown that the risk is reduced by only about 2%. Carotid endarterectomy carries a 1% risk of mortality and a 2% risk of intraoperative neurological deficit.

Indications for carotid artery Doppler imaging include: TIA; amaurosis fugax; carotid bruit; preoperative assessment follow-up endarterectomy; and patients at risk of vascular disease. Also studies have shown that an intima-medial thickness (IMT) in the CCA of more than 0.8 mm can predict individuals at risk of developing atheroma at other sites and this has become a screening tool.

A number of measurements are used for the assessment of the degree of carotid artery stenosis: peak systolic velocity (PSV) in the CCA; PSV in the ICA; ICA end-diastolic velocity (EDV); and the PSV ratio of ICA/CCA. For example, a greater than 70% diameter stenosis at the origin of the internal carotid artery would give an ICA PSV of > 230 cm/s, an ICA EDV of > 75 cm/s, and an ICA/CCA PSV ratio of > 3.

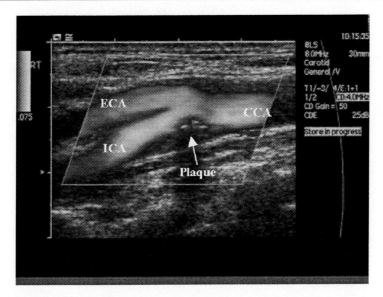

Fig. 37b   Carotid Doppler ultrasound image showing a plaque in the carotid bulb, extending into the origin of the internal carotid artery (ICA), resulting in a stenosis. CCA, Common carotid artery; ECA, external carotid artery.

Question 38

A 66-year-old man presented with a depressed Glasgow coma scale after a fall downstairs. What abnormalities are present on the plain film skull series (Figs 38a, b, and c)?

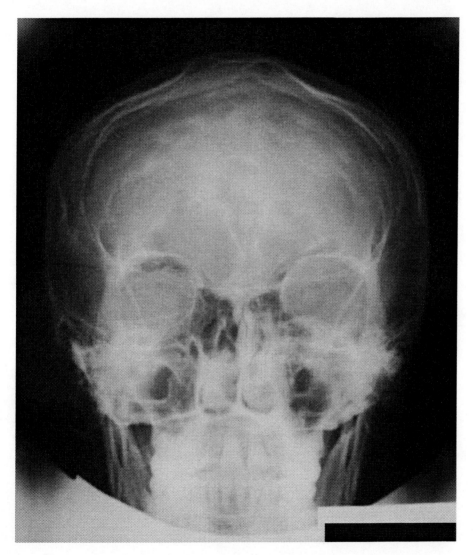

Fig. 38a

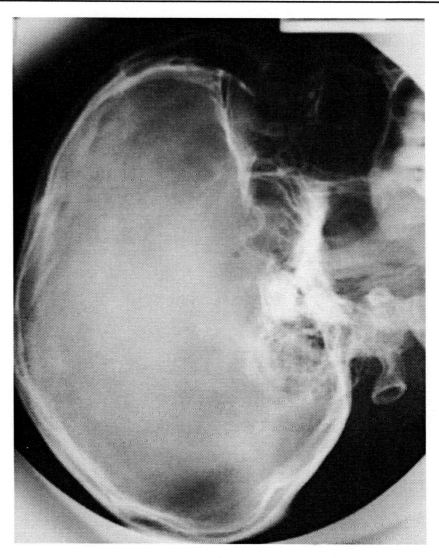

Fig. 38b

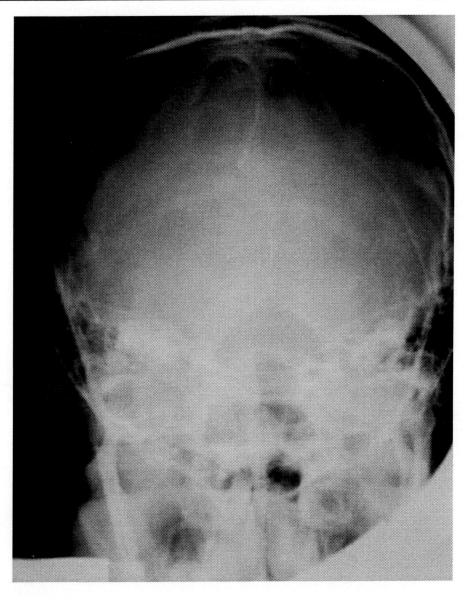

Fig. 38c

Answer 38

Findings: The frontal facial view (Fig. 38d) shows periorbital emphysema (arrow).

On the lateral horizontal beam film (Fig. 38e; taken with the patient lying supine) an air–fluid level (arrow) is present in the sphenoid sinus consistent with blood. In addition, intracranial air (arrowheads) is present (projected over the temporal bone).

On the Towne's view (Fig. 38f) there is a right occipital fracture (arrows). The patient had periorbital ecchymosis ('racoon eyes') consistent with a basal skull fracture (not shown).

The presence of intracranial air is indicative of a fracture involving the paranasal sinuses (sphenoid, maxillary, frontal, and ethmoid) or mastoid sinuses. Orbital emphysema results from a fracture that allows communication with the adjacent paranasal sinuses. The weakest part of the orbital margin is medially—the thin lamina papyracea bone. Intracranial air is also seen in fractures of the base of skull. Often, only tiny volumes of air, which are much easier to visualize on 'lung' CT windows than on bone or brain windows, enter the cranium. Air is most often seen in the non-dependent portion of the cranium anterior to the frontal lobes or adjacent to the falx. Blood seen in the sinuses, nasal cavity, mastoids, middle ear, or external auditory canal is the other sign of base of skull fractures. Visualizing the basal skull fracture itself can be difficult, and fine thickness cuts may be helpful. The sphenoid bone is involved in 15% of skull-base fractures and may be complicated by cerebrospinal fluid (CSF) rhinorrhoea/otorrhoea indicative of a dural tear. The majority of these resolve spontaneously but, if there is a persistent CSF leak, water-soluble intrathecal contrast material is useful in demonstrating a fistula.

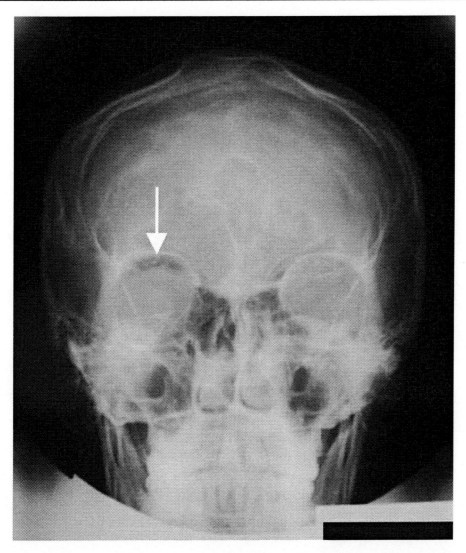

Fig. 38d   The frontal facial view shows periorbital emphysema (arrow).

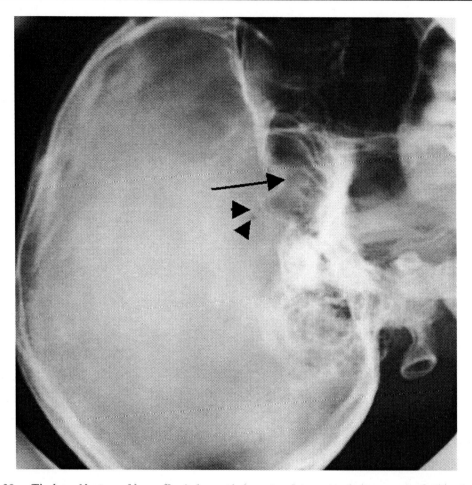

Fig. 38e   *The lateral horizontal beam film (taken with the patient lying supine) shows an air–fluid level (arrow) in the sphenoid sinus, consistent with blood. Intracranial air (arrowheads) is also present (projected over the temporal bone).*

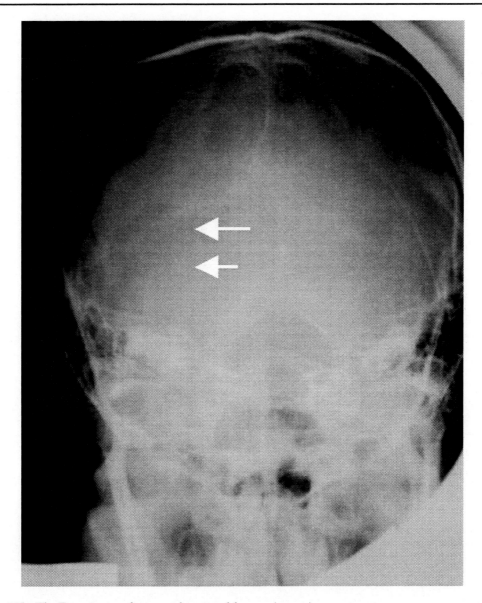

Fig. 38f   The Towne's view shows a right occipital fracture (arrows).

Question 39

A 24-year-old was brought to casualty having been assaulted. A facial view is shown (Fig. 39). What abnormality is present? What was the patient's presenting complaint?

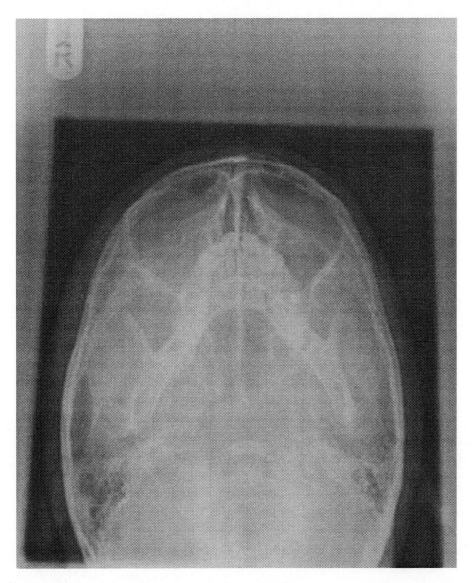

Fig. 39

Answer 39: Blow-out fracture of orbital floor

Findings: There is a blow-out fracture of the right inferior orbital floor with inferior herniation of orbital contents (inferior rectus and inferior oblique muscles). The herniated material is seen as opacification of the right maxillary antrum.

Patients may complain of diplopia on upward gaze.

Blow-out fractures are caused by a direct blow to the globe with a resultant sudden increase in intraorbital pressure that is transmitted to the orbital floor. Fracture of the delicate lamina papyracea bone often occurs. A direct hit on the globe by a squash ball is a classic history. Herniation of orbital fat or of the inferior extra-ocular eye muscles, which become entrapped resulting in diplopia on upward gaze, may occur. This is an indication for surgical correction. Posttraumatic atrophy of orbital fat may lead to enophthalmus.

Question 40

What abnormalities are present on this postoperative chest X-ray (Fig. 40)? What action should be suggested?

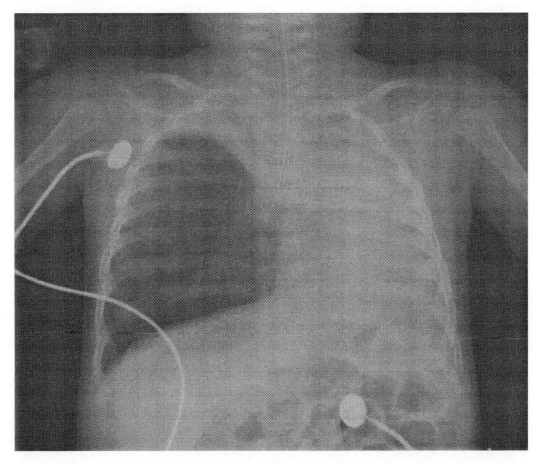

Fig. 40

Answer 40

The abnormalities are:

- complete collapse of the left lung;
- right upper lobe collapse;
- the tip of the endotracheal tube (ETT) is erroneously sited in the bronchus intermedius.

The ETT should be withdrawn so that its tip lies above the carina. Physiotherapy, tracheal suction, and/or ventilation may be necessary to aid reinflation.

Findings: There is complete opacification of the left hemithorax with loss of volume, seen as mediastinal shift to the left and elevation of the left hemidiaphragm. In the right upper zone there is an area of increased density bounded inferiorly by the right horizontal fissure, which has been displaced superiorly. This is the appearance of a right upper lobe collapse. The right hilum is elevated and there is compensatory hyperinflation of the right lower lobe, which is more translucent than normal.

Collapse is denoted by opacity and volume loss on a chest radiograph. On a normal chest X-ray (CXR) the mediastinal contour and left hemidiaphragm are seen silhouetted against the normally aerated left lung. If there is collapse of the left lung these structures are no longer seen due to loss of the silhouette sign (there is no longer differential photon absorption between air in the lung and soft tissue of the mediastinum, so the collapsed lobe and adjacent mediastinal soft tissue appear white on the X-ray film).

The most common causes of collapse are pneumonia, mucous plugging (asthma and cystic fibrosis), bronchial neoplasm, and inhaled foreign body.

On a CXR the basic features of lobar collapse are opacity and loss of volume. The resulting signs are:

- increased density of pulmonary tissue;
- completely obscured pulmonary vessels;
- effacement of normally identified interfaces between air within the lung and surrounding soft tissues (silhouette sign);
- displacement of fissures;
- displacement of the hilum towards the collapse;
- movement of bronchi and blood vessels (crowding in the affected lobe and splaying in the normal lobes on the same side);
- elevation of the hemidiaphragm;
- shift of the mediastinum (heart and/or trachea) towards the side of collapse;
- compensatory hyperinflation of normal lung.

Question 41

This 66-year-old man presented with haemoptysis and dyspnoea. What does the chest radiograph (Fig. 41a) show?

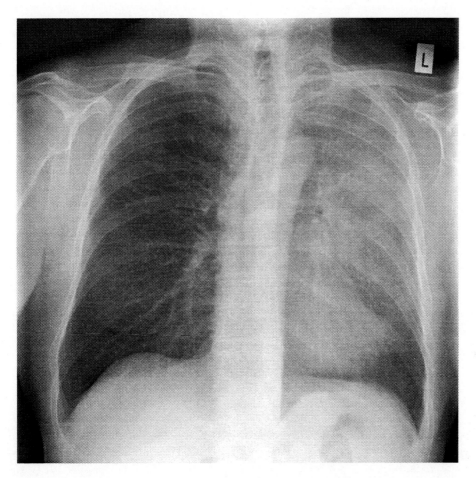

Fig. 41a

Answer 41: Left upper lobe collapse secondary to a bronchogenic carcinoma

Findings: There is a veil-like opacity over the left hemithorax with obscuration of the left heart border. There is volume loss with elevation of the left hemidiaphragm. An area of increased density is seen at the left hilum, likely to be a mass consistent with a bronchial cancer.

Figure 41b shows an enhanced CT scan in the same patient at the level of the carina. There is a bronchial cancer (straight arrows) obstructing the origin of the left upper lobe bronchus, causing distal collapse (arrowheads). Pathological subcarinal lymphadenopathy (LN) is seen. There is also a pulmonary embolus in the right main pulmonary artery (open arrow). CT is useful in staging bronchial cancer and assessing operability.

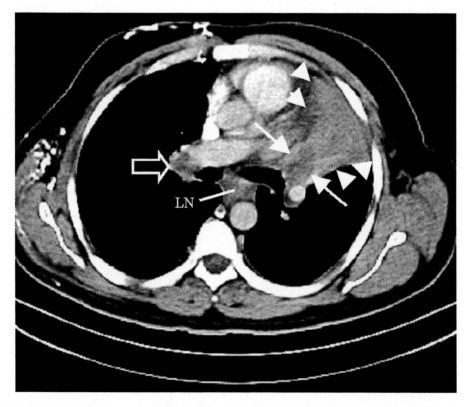

Fig. 41b   An enhanced CT scan at the level of the carina showing a bronchial cancer (straight arrows) obstructing the origin of the left upper lobe bronchus, causing distal collapse (arrowheads). Pathological subcarinal lymphadenopathy (LN) is also seen and there is a pulmonary embolus in the right main pulmonary artery (open arrow).

Question 42

This elderly demented patient presented with gross abdominal distension. What does the abdominal film (Fig. 42a) show?

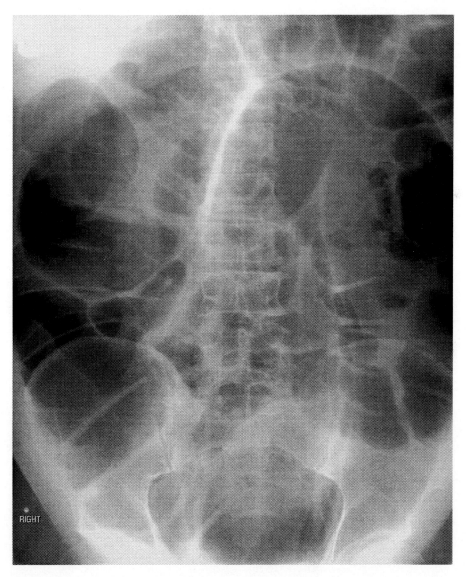

Fig. 42a

Answer 42: Sigmoid volvulus

Findings: There is a markedly distended loop of bowel arising from the pelvis and extending superiorly to the left upper quadrant. The loop has the appearance of a coffee bean. There are absent haustral markings in the loop. The appearances are consistent with a sigmoid volvulus. The proximal large bowel is dilated in keeping with obstruction.

In sigmoid volvulus the colon twists on its mesenteric axis. The condition is common in African and Asian countries due to their high fibre diet. In the West the patients are commonly elderly, or psychiatric cases. The sigmoid becomes a greatly distended, paralysed loop and this is described on plain abdominal X-rays as having the appearance of a 'coffee bean'. The midline crease corresponds to the mesenteric root. The diagnosis may be confirmed by a water-soluble contrast enema, which shows a 'bird's beak' deformity (Fig. 42b) at the point of volvulus (rectosigmoid junction). The CT manifestation of this appearance is tightly coiled vessels, mesentery, and bowel at the site of the volvulus.

Acute management can commonly be with decompression using a flatus tube. As the condition commonly recurs, surgical intervention may be needed to fix or excise the offending loop.

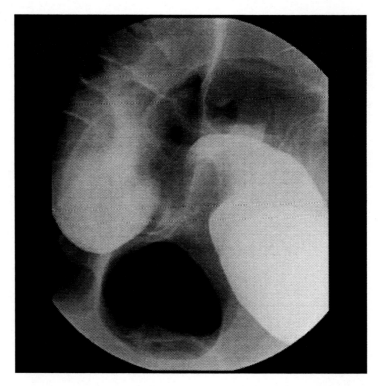

Fig. 42b   Contrast enema showing a 'bird's beak' deformity at the apex of a sigmoid volvulus.

Question 43

This 26-year-old year man injured his knee (Fig. 43) whilst skiing. What is the injury called? What associated injuries should be excluded?

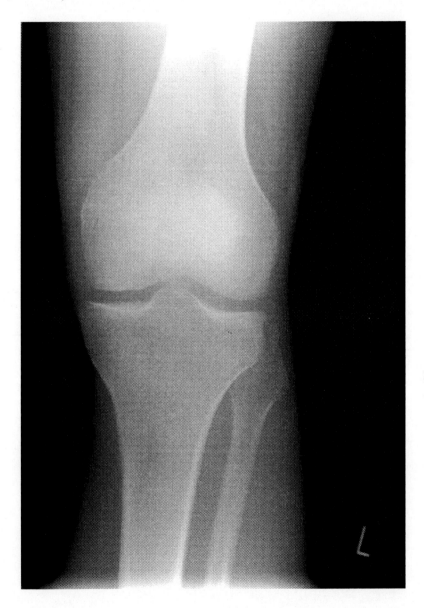

Fig. 43

Answer 43: Segond fracture

This fracture is associated with anterior cruciate ligament (ACL) and lateral meniscal tears.

Findings: There is a bony fragment lateral to the lateral tibial plateau consistent with a cortical avulsion fracture of the proximal lateral tibial plateau.

A Segond fracture is an avulsion injury at the insertion of the middle third of the lateral capsular ligament on the upper lateral tibia. ACL tears are associated in 75–100%, and lateral meniscal tears in 67% of cases. This may result in chronic anterolateral knee instability. The mechanism of injury is due to internal rotation associated with varus stress on a flexed knee causing tension of the lateral capsular ligament. A tear of the capsule and avulsion of the fibular head by lateral collateral ligament avulsion may also occur.

Question 44

This 34-year-old man was referred for a cardiothoracic opinion following the discovery of a lung lesion on a routine insurance chest radiograph (Fig. 44a). A CT was then performed (Fig. 44b). What do the investigations show? What is the diagnosis?

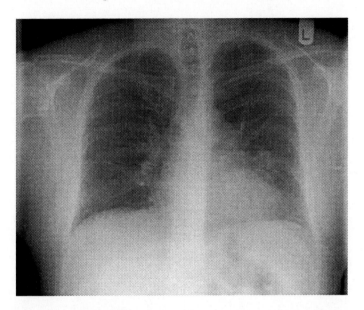

Fig. 44a

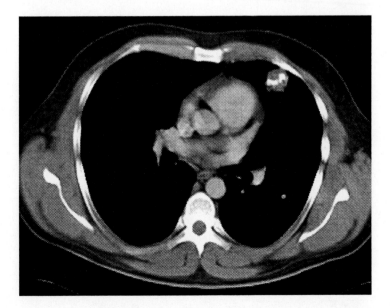

Fig. 44b

Answer 44: Pulmonary hamartoma

Findings: The chest radiograph shows a well-defined lesion abutting the left heart border (therefore in the lingual segment). On close inspection 'popcorn' calcification is seen in the lesion. The CT confirms the presence of central popcorn calcification typical of a pulmonary hamartoma.

A hamartoma is a mass composed of tissues normally found in that organ, but in an abnormal quantity and arrangement. A pulmonary hamartoma is the most common benign lung tumour. Hamartomas are usually picked up in the fifth and sixth decade and are mostly asymptomatic. Hamartomas may present with haemoptysis or infection (post-obstructive pneumonitis). They are characteristically round, smooth, lobulated masses less than 4 cm in size of which 66% are peripheral and 10% endobronchial. Popcorn calcification is seen in 15% of hamartomas and is virtually pathognomonic. Fat is present in 50% on CT. They may grow slowly and occasionally still require resection.

Question 45

This 53-year-old patient presented with abdominal pain. What does the Doppler ultrasound of the right upper quadrant show (Fig. 45a)?

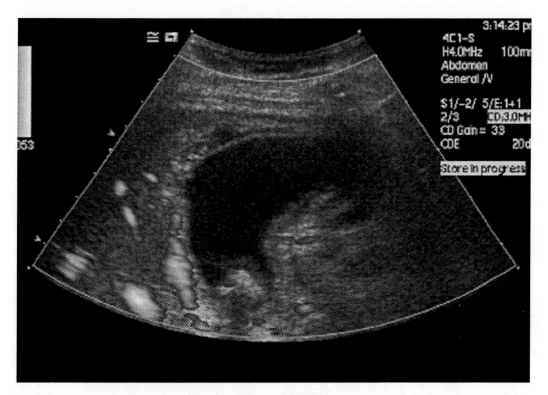

Fig. 45a

Answer 45: Acute cholecystitis

Findings: The ultrasound shows a thick-walled gallbladder with a gallstone in the neck. There is increased Doppler signal in the gallbladder wall indicative of inflammatory hyper-vascularity.

Acute cholecystitis occurs because of cystic duct obstruction by a calculus in 90% of cases. Females are affected three times as commonly as males and the condition most frequently presents between the ages of 40 and 60 years.

Patients present with right upper quadrant pain (which often radiates to the right shoulder region), nausea, vomiting, and fever and, on examination, there is right upper quadrant tenderness and guarding.

Ultrasound is the initial examination of choice in diagnosis (sensitivity 85–94%). Ultrasound signs include: gallbladder wall thickening (> 3 mm), 'splitting' of the gallbladder wall with an echopoor oedematous middle layer, a poorly defined gallbladder wall, debris in the bile (due to pus, blood, or sludge), increased colour Doppler flow in the gallbladder wall, and pericholecystic fluid. Gallstones are identified in more than 90% of cases and a calculus is commonly seen impacted in the gallbladder neck. In cases of diagnostic difficulty, nuclear medicine imaging, or magnetic resonance imaging can be used for problem solving.

Complications of acute cholecystitis include gangrene of the gallbladder, perforation of the gallbladder (2–20%), emphysematous cholecystitis (Fig. 45b), and empyema of the gallbladder.

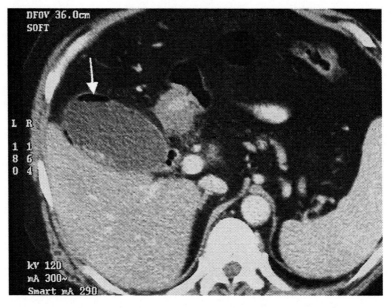

Fig. 45b   Gas is present in the gallbladder (arrow) in a case of emphysematous cholecystitis.

Question 46

This 56-year-old lady presented with lower abdominal pain and distension. What does the abdominal radiograph (Fig. 46) show?

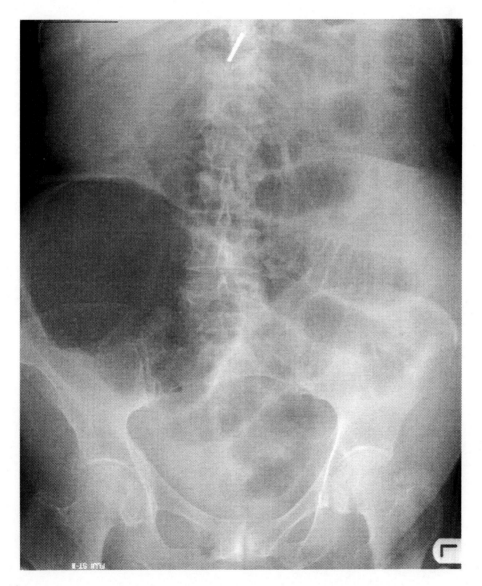

Fig. 46

Answer 46: Caecal volvulus

Findings: There is a large dilated loop of bowel with a thickened wall in the right iliac fossa. The rest of the colon is not dilated. The appearances are consistent with a caecal volvulus. There is small bowel obstruction.

Caecal volvulus is associated with malrotation and a long caecal mesentery. The condition is more common in men and the peak age of presentation is 20–40 years.

On the plain abdominal radiograph the volvulus appears as 'kidney-shaped' distension of the caecum, commonly positioned in the left upper quadrant. Barium enema demonstrates tapering of the barium column towards the torsion. CT demonstrates the distended caecum and the point of torsion. Depending upon the competency of the ileocaecal valve, there may be associated small bowel distension. Caecal volvulus may arise secondary to a distal obstructing lesion, e.g. carcinoma.

Question 47

This 82-year-old patient presented with pain and jaundice. What investigation is shown (Fig. 47)? What is the diagnosis?

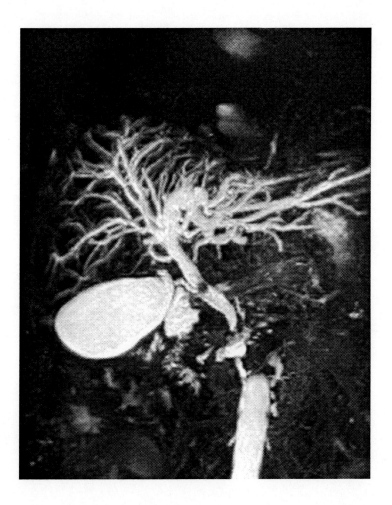

Fig. 47

Answer 47: Magnetic resonance cholangiopancreatogram (MRCP)

A calculus in the common bile duct (seen as a filling defect)

Gallstones are the most common cause of bile duct obstruction, being responsible in about 75% of cases. Bile duct calculi should be considered in patients with a recent history of jaundice, a recent history of pancreatitis, elevated bilirubin, elevated amylase, and where the bile duct is dilated. The patients often report recurrent episodes of jaundice, with associated fever.

Ultrasound is the first modality of choice for imaging biliary calculi, but stones may be missed due to overlying bowel gas and in non-dilated systems. The investigation of choice for common bile duct calculus is MRCP. The sensitivity and specificity of this investigation are in excess of 90%. This significantly outperforms both CT and ultrasound (sensitivity 50%) and is without the risks associated with endoscopic retrograde cholangiopancreatography (ERCP). Heavily T2-weighted (showing fluid as high signal in the ducts and bowel) sequences are acquired during a single breathhold. Stones < 6 mm in size may pass spontaneously. However, ERCP may be required to remove larger stones. This carries a risk of pancreatitis and, if sphincterotomy is performed, of haemorrhage.

Question 48

This 65-year-old long-stay inpatient presented with a 2-day history of bloody diarrhoea and increasing abdominal pain. What does the plain abdominal radiograph (Fig. 48) show? List three causes.

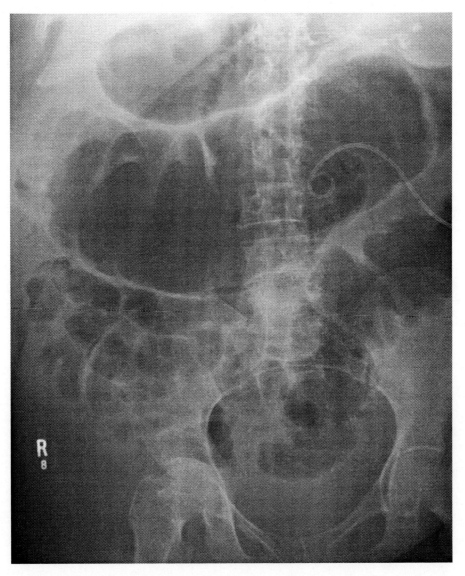

Fig. 48

Answer 48: Toxic megacolon

Possible causes are ulcerative colitis, Crohn's disease, pseudomembranous colitis, ischaemia, bacillary dysentery, amoebiasis, typhoid fever, cholera, and Behçet's disease.

Findings: There is marked dilatation of the transverse colon with thickening of the bowel wall caused by mucosal oedema. The maximum transverse colonic diameter is 12 cm (upper limit of normal 5.5 cm). No intramural or free intraperitoneal air is seen. A left nephrostomy is *in situ*. This patient developed pseudomembranous colitis after a long inpatient stay with multiple courses of antibiotics.

Toxic megacolon is due to transmural fulminant colitis with neuromuscular degeneration. This results in rapid colon dilatation. Typically there is loss of the normal haustral pattern with bowel wall thickening and pseudopolyposis (mucosal islands in denuded ulcerated colonic wall). It is important to differentiate toxic megacolon from other causes of a dilated colon where the mucosal pattern will be normal, e.g. ileus, pseudoobstruction, and true obstruction. As well as the radiological findings, the diagnosis is also based on the patient's clinical condition, i.e. the presence of pyrexia, tachycardia, and leucocytosis. Perforation and ensuing peritonitis may occur with a high mortality (> 20%). Perforation may be heralded by linear air within the bowel wall. Sigmoidoscopy and rectal biopsy usually yield the underlying cause, but a barium enema is contraindicated.

Question 49

This barium enema (Fig. 49) was performed on a 26-year-old man with altered bowel habit. What is the diagnosis?

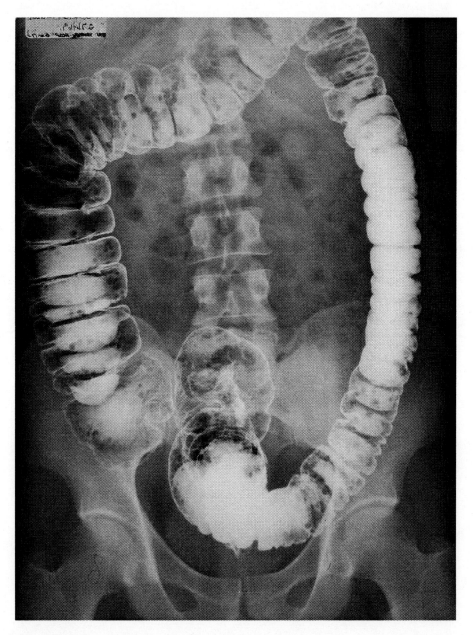

Fig. 49

Answer 49: Cancer of the sigmoid colon complicating familial polyposis coli

Findings: The colon is carpeted with small polyps. There is an annular stenosing lesion in the sigmoid colon consistent with a carcinoma.

Familial adenomatous polyposis coli is an autosomal dominant disease (due to an abnormality of the adenomatous polyposis (APC) gene on chromosome 5) with 80% penetration. The condition occurs sporadically in one-third. Polyps appear around the second or third decade of life, causing rectal bleeding, diarrhoea, and mucus discharge.

The colon is affected in all patients with development of carcinoma at a rate of 30% after 10 years, and 100% after 20 years. There is a high proportion (80%) of multifocal carcinomas. A prophylactic proctocolectomy is therefore performed once the condition is diagnosed. Relatives should be screened by colonoscopy from their early teens to middle age.

The condition is also associated with hamartomas of the stomach (50%), adenomas of the duodenum (25%), desmoid tumours, papillary thyroid carcinoma, and periampullary carcinoma.

Gardner's syndrome is a variant of this condition. In addition to the colonic adenomas, upper gastrointestinal malignancies, skull osteomata, epidermoid cysts, desmoid tumours, and dental abnormalities may be found.

Question 50

This 54-year-old patient had a history of altered bowel habit. A barium enema was performed (Fig. 50). What is the diagnosis? What underlying conditions are associated with this appearance?

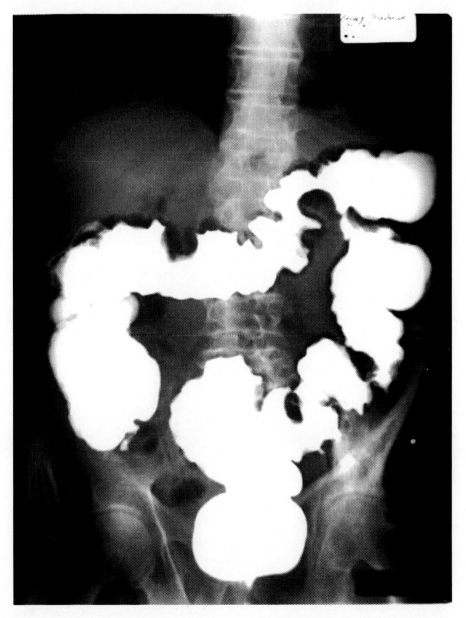

Fig. 50

Answer 50: Pneumatosis coli

Associated conditions are chronic obstructive airways disease, asthma, connective tissue diseases (scleroderma, polymyositis), peptic ulceration, intestinal bypass surgery, postendoscopy, and, rarely, inflammatory bowel disease.

Findings: There are widespread radiolucent lesions along the contour of the colon consistent with submucosal gas cysts characteristic of pneumatosis coli.

In pneumatosis coli (pneumatosis cystoides intestinalis) nitrogen cysts occur in the submucosal and subserosal layers of the bowel wall. They are usually on the mesenteric side of the bowel. They may rupture resulting in pneumoperitoneum without peritonitis. Recognition of pneumatosis coli as the underlying cause is essential to avoid unnecessary laparotomy. Pneumatosis coli is most common in the sigmoid and descending colon.

Patients are usually asymptomatic but may present with vague abdominal pain, diarrhoea, or constipation. Treatment is usually unnecessary, but if the patient is symptomatic hyperbaric oxygen therapy may be used. Since the gas in the cyst is predominantly nitrogen, oxygen therapy lowers the partial pressure of other gases in the blood so facilitating diffusion of nitrogen from the cysts. In contrast to pneumatosis coli, the presence of linear intramural gas is a sinister sign of bowel necrosis/infarction.

Question 51

This patient had a long history of abdominal pain and weight loss. An image from a barium follow-through examination is shown (Fig. 51a). What is the most likely diagnosis?

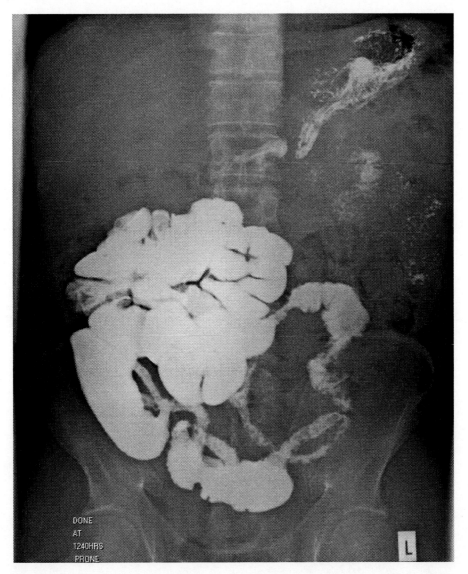

Fig. 51a

Answer 51: Crohn's disease

Findings: There are multiple skip lesions with ulcerated strictured small bowel segments. There is a small bowel enteroenteric fistula on the left side of the abdomen (at the site of convergence of bowel loops). The proximal small bowel is dilated consistent with a partial obstruction. Separation of the affected bowel loops is present due to wall thickening and inflammation as well as mesenteric fibrofatty proliferation.

Crohn's disease most commonly affects the small bowel. Small bowel barium findings are of thickened and nodular folds, aphthous ulcers, cobblestone mucosa, and deep 'rose-thorn' ulceration, 'skip areas' of involvement, and strictures.

Complications include abscesses (Fig. 51b), fistulae, mesenteric lymphadenopathy, fibrofatty proliferation of the mesentery, toxic megacolon, and an increased incidence of adenocarcinoma and lymphoma.

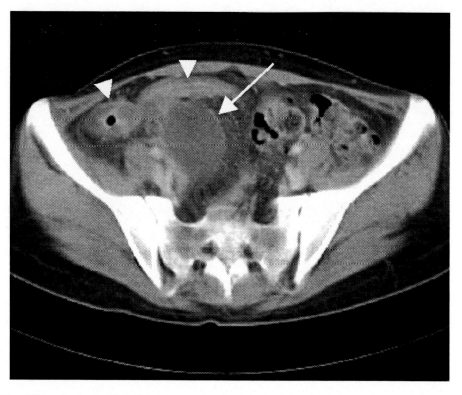

Fig. 51b   CT section in another patient showing a pelvic abscess (arrow) adjacent to thickened bowel loops (arrowheads) in Crohn's disease.

Question 52

A 26-year-old known haemophiliac was admitted with severe right loin pain. The abdominal radiograph (Fig. 52a) is shown. What abnormality is present on the abdominal radiograph?

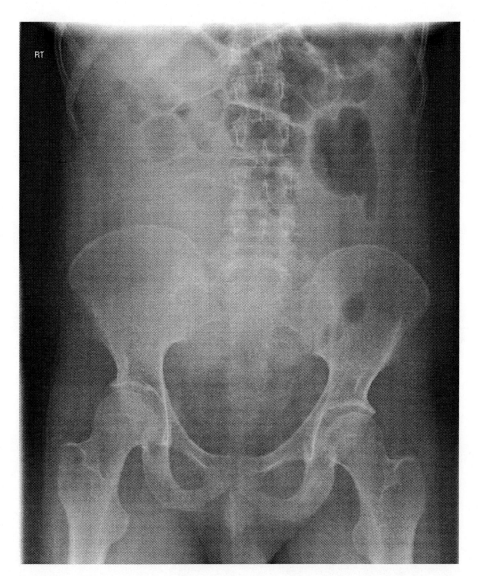

Fig. 52a

Answer 52: Right psoas haematoma

Findings: The abdominal film demonstrates loss of the normal right psoas silhouette sign with increased density over the right flank consistent with retroperitoneal pathology. There is a scoliosis of the lumbar spine, concave to the right, due to associated muscular spasm. Note the normal left psoas margin (interface between fat and muscle).

The CT (Fig. 52b) shows a right intrapsoas haematoma (arrow) with stranding in the adjacent fat.

The differential diagnosis for retroperitoneal lesions includes:

1   haemorrhage:
    •   patients with a coagulopathy or on anticoagulants;
    •   trauma;
    •   leaking aortic aneurysms;
2   neoplastic:
    •   primary sarcoma or lymphoma; metastases from breast or bronchus carcinoma;
3   retroperitoneal fibrosis;
4   infections arising from:
    •   tuberculosis (or other organisms, such as brucellosis or streptococcus) from adjacent discitis or osteomyelitis. This may present as a psoas abscess;
    •   renal abscesses/pyleonephritis;
    •   pancreatic/appendiceal/intestinal pathologies such as Crohn's disease.

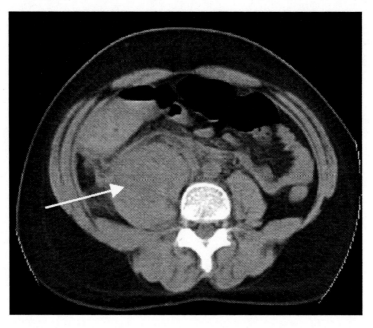

Fig. 52b   CT of the same patient showing a right intrapsoas haematoma (arrow) with stranding in the adjacent fat.

Question 53

This 36-year-old patient had a past history of retroperitoneal haemorrhage. An image from a selective renal angiogram (Fig. 53a) is shown. What abnormalities are present? What is the diagnosis?

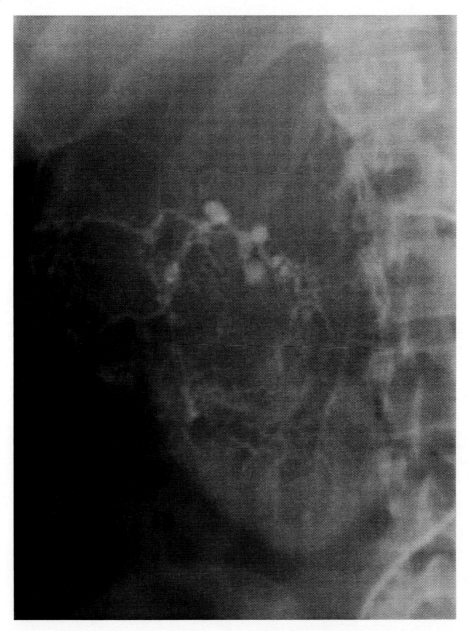

Fig. 53a

Answer 53: Renal angiomyolipoma

The angiogram shows a vascular mass arising from the upper pole of the right kidney extending beyond the normal cortical contour. The mass is of reduced density suggestive of the presence of fat in the lesion. Multiple microaneurysms are present. Note the normally enhancing lower renal pole.

A renal angiomyolipoma (AML) is a hamartoma, histologically composed of fat, smooth muscle, and tortuous irregular aneurysmal arteries. Eighty per cent are sporadic. These are usually unilateral and more common in females between 40 and 60 years of age. Twenty per cent of AMLs occur in tuberous sclerosis (TS) (80% of TS patients have AMLs). This is an autosomally dominant inherited neuroectodermal disorder characterized by central nervous system hamartomas, fits, cutaneous adenoma sebaceum (epiloia), subungual fibromata, retinal phakomata, and mental retardation.

Small AMLs are asymptomatic. There is an increased risk of haemorrhage in lesions greater than 4 cm in size. Shock may occur from haemorrhage from the microaneuryms into the AML or the retroperitoneum. AMLs larger than 4 cm may therefore require nephrectomy or embolization. The characteristic fat lucency of AMLs can be seen on plain films and CT (Fig. 53b). On ultrasound AMLs are echogenic (due to their fat content). High signal is seen on T1-weighted MR sequences.

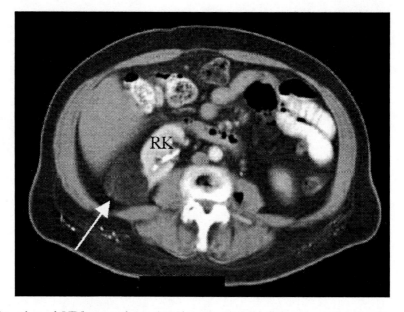

Fig 53b An enhanced CT from another patient shows an angiomyolipoma (arrow) arising from the right kidney (RK). The lesion is mainly composed of fat as its attenuation is similar to that of the adjacent mesenteric fat.

Question 54

This 63-year-old lady underwent an intravenous urogram (IVU; Fig. 54) for investigation of painless haematuria. What abnormalities are present? What is the differential diagnosis for these appearances?

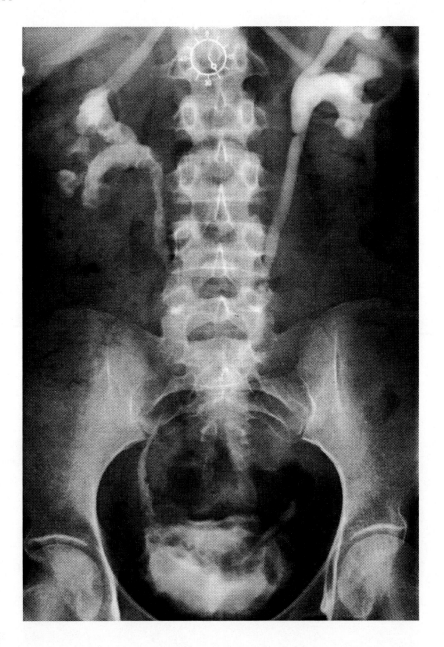

Fig. 54

Answer 54: Pyeloureteritis cystica

Findings: Multifocal, small, round lucent defects (crazy paving appearance) are seen in the right pelvicalyceal system, right ureter, and bladder. The diagnosis was pyeloureteritis cystica.

The differential diagnosis for these appearances is:

- multifocal transitional cell carcinoma;
- malacoplakia;
- multifocal submucosal haemorrhage;
- multiple polyps;
- allergic mucosal urticaria.

Pyeloureteritis cystica is due to multifocal submucosal oedema, which form as a result of chronic urinary tract irritation secondary to infection or calculi. There is an increased incidence in diabetics. The most common organisms are *E. coli*, mycobacterium tuberculosis, *Proteus enterococcus*, and schistosomiasis. The abnormality may persist for years in spite of antibiotic therapy. The bladder is most commonly affected, followed by the proximal one-third of the ureter. The condition is usually unilateral. The most important differential diagnosis is multifocal transitional cell carcinoma.

Question 55

What injury has this 27-year-old man sustained (Fig. 55)?

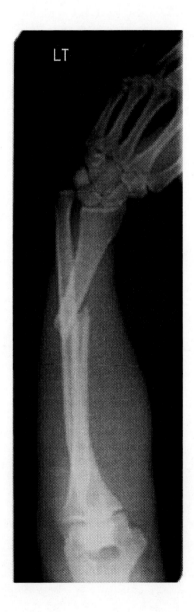

Fig. 55

Answer 55: Galeazzi fracture

Findings: There is a fracture of the distal left radius with dislocation of the distal radioulnar joint.

The mechanism of injury in a Galeazzi fracture is a fall on an outstretched hand with hyperpronation of the forearm. Treatment is reduction and internal fixation. There is a high incidence of non-union, delayed union, and malunion.

Question 56

This 28-year-old lady underwent an uncomplicated appendicectomy for acute appendicitis. Ten days postoperatively she re-presented with fever, vomiting, and upper abdominal pain. What does the contrast-enhanced CT (Fig. 56) show?

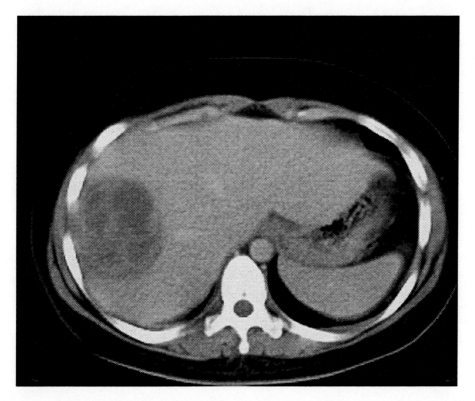

Fig. 56

Answer 56: Pyogenic liver abscess

Findings: In the right lobe of liver there is a rim-enhancing, multiloculated, focal hypodensity consistent with an abscess.

Pyogenic liver abscesses are uncommon. The underlying cause may be: ascending cholangitis (the most common cause, with multiple abscess found in over 90%); portal phlebitis (secondary to an infective focus within the drainage area of the portal vein); pyogenic hepatic arterial emboli; extension from an adjacent septic process; or traumatic introduction of septic material. Abscess formation from appendicitis and diverticulitis is now rare. In adults the most common organism isolated is *Strep. milleri* and in children it is *Staph. aureus*. Ultrasound is usually the initial imaging modality used. The ultrasound features are variable, but scanning of a liquefied abscess commonly shows a well-defined hypoechoic lesion, with a mildly hyperechoic rim and distal enhancement. There may be debris within the abscess, and strongly echogenic foci resulting from gas are seen in 20% of cases. The sensitivity for lesions varies with size, but is up to 90% for 15 mm abscesses. If the abscess is scanned in the pre-liquefaction stage it appears as solid echopoor lesion. CT has a sensitivity of over 95%. The abscess is usually shown as a rounded, well-defined, hypodense lesion with a peripheral rim that enhances after the administration of intravenous contrast. In some cases, septation or a cluster of cavities is seen.

Treatment is with drainage, where possible via an image-guided, percutaneous route, and antibiotics. The underlying cause must be identified.

Question 57

This 40-year-old male presented with itching and right upper quadrant pain. What abnormalities are present on the endoscopic retrograde cholangiopancreatogram (ERCP; Fig. 57)? What is the diagnosis?

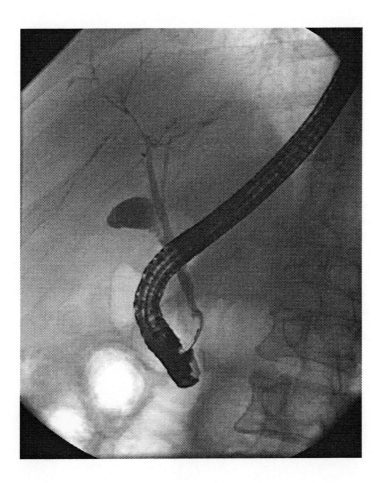

Fig. 57

Answer 57: Sclerosing cholangitis

Findings: There are multiple strictures causing irregularity of the calibre of the biliary tree, which result in a 'beaded' appearance.

Primary sclerosing cholangitis (PSC) affects males twice as often as females and most patients are under 45 years at the age of presentation. Secondary sclerosing cholangitis is associated with inflammatory bowel disease (70% have ulcerative colitis), cirrhosis, chronic active hepatitis, pancreatitis, retroperitoneal fibrosis, and thyroiditis. Patients present with: chronic intermittent jaundice, fatigue, pruritus, right upper quadrant pain, and fever (30%). There is usually an elevated serum alkaline phosphatase, with mildly abnormal bilirubin and transaminase levels.

Histologically, the strictures result from non-uniform chronic obliterative inflammatory fibrosis. Areas of ductal normality exist between the ductal strictures, and duct dilatation may be present upstream from strictures. The combination of strictures and dilatation gives the 'beaded' appearance typical of PSC. The differential diagnosis includes cholangio-carcinoma (marked duct dilatation upstream from a dominant stricture), acute ascending cholangitis (the history should allow differentiation), and primary biliary cirrhosis (the disease is usually limited to the intrahepatic biliary tree).

Imaging is required to establish a firm diagnosis in many cases. ERCP and magnetic resonance cholangiopancreatography (MRCP) are the most sensitive and specific modalities. Strictures vary in length from 1 mm to several cm. The common bile duct is almost always involved, and the intra- and extrahepatic ducts are involved in combination in up to 90% of patients. Involvement of the gall bladder is seen in 15%. As the process progresses, peripheral ducts become obliterated and the appearance of the biliary tree is that of a 'pruned tree'. There may be 'diverticula' up to 10 mm in size (25%).

CT and ultrasound demonstrate the features identified on ERCP and MRCP but with less precision, although the advantages are that they demonstrate the entire biliary tree when duct filling at ERCP may be prevented by strictures; and they identify the complications of PSC (cirrhosis, portal hypertension, and cholangiocarcinoma).

Question 58

This 79-year-old patient presented with recurrent episodes of right upper quadrant pain followed by an acute episode of abdominal distension with vomiting. What abnormalities have been arrowed on the film (Fig. 58a)? What is the diagnosis?

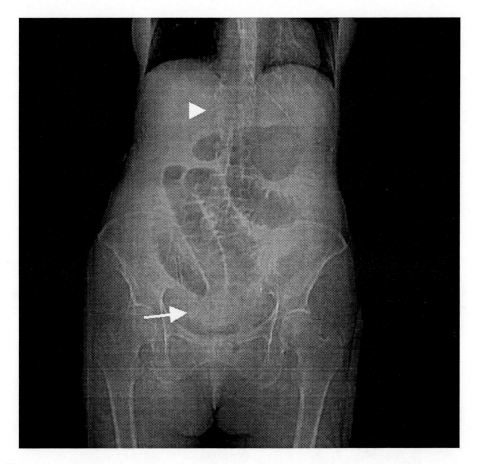

Fig. 58a

Answer 58: Gallstone ileus

Findings: The abnormalities are aerobilia (air in the biliary tree denoted by arrowhead) and an ectopic gallstone in the distal small bowel (arrow).

The above abnormalities along with the presence of small bowel obstruction (dilated small bowel loops) are pathognomonic of gallstone ileus (Rigler's triad).

Patients with gallstone ileus commonly present with a past history of gallbladder disease, intermittent acute colicky abdominal pain, nausea, vomiting, fever, and distension. The most common age range is 65–75 years and females are affected five times as often as males.

Gallstone ileus is an uncommon cause of intestinal obstruction (about 1%) but has a high mortality. However, with increasing age it becomes a more likely cause of intestinal obstruction (25% in patients over 70 years). The gallstone enters the small bowel via a fistula. This is most commonly cholecystoduodenal (60%) and results in aerobilia seen as a branching lucencies arising from the liver hilum in contrast to the peripheral air present with portal venous gas. The gallstone needs to be larger than 2.5 cm to cause small bowel obstruction. The gallstone most commonly impacts in the terminal ileum (60–70%).

The classic plain radiograph triad is intestinal obstruction (80%), gas in the biliary tree (70%), and an ectopic calcified gallstone (25%). Comparison with old abdominal radiographs is often useful, as the gallstone will usually have been present previously and shows a change in position when compared with the new film.

CT is often the best diagnostic test. It can confirm the small bowel obstruction; identify the ectopic gallstone (Fig. 58b) and the fistulous communication as well as the gas in the biliary tree with greater sensitivity than a plain radiograph or ultrasound. Surgical relief of the obstruction is necessary via an enterotomy.

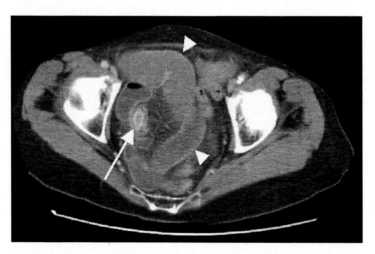

Fig 58b   CT section through the pelvis showing dilated loops of small bowel (arrowheads) and an ectopic gallstone (arrow) impacted in the terminal ileum consistent with gallstone ileus.

Question 59

This 33-year-old man had a history of recurrent urinary tract infections. What abnormality is demonstrated on the intravenous urogram (IVU; Fig. 59)? What is the diagnosis?

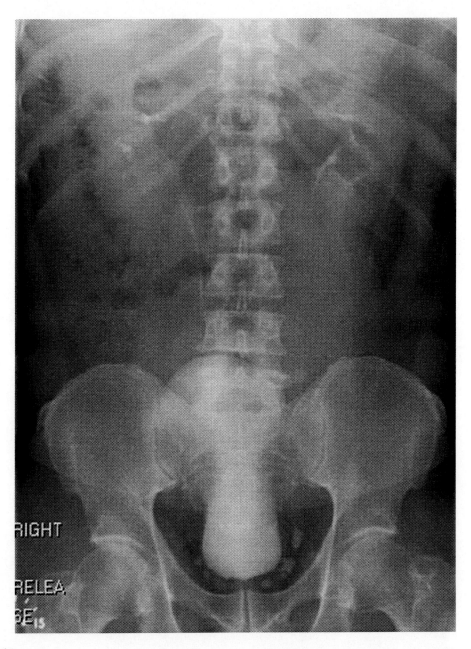

Fig. 59

Answer 59: Pelvic lipomatosis

Findings: There is elongation and elevation of the bladder resulting in 'an inverted pear shape'. There is also perivesical lucency suggestive of increased pelvic fat deposition. The upper renal tracts are normal.

Pelvic lipomatosis is a non-malignant overgrowth of adipose tissue that causes compression of pelvic structures. There may be an associated inflammatory and fibrotic component. Pelvic lipomatosis is more common in males (male:female 10:1) but is not associated with obesity. Patients may present with urinary frequency and loin and back pain as well as urinary tract infections due to failure to completely empty the bladder. The rectum is also narrowed and the sigmoid colon is elevated out of the pelvis. Complications include ureteric and inferior vena cava (IVC) obstruction.

Question 60

This 64-year-old man presented with right renal colic. What abnormalities do the unenhanced CT sections through the kidneys (Fig. 60a) and bladder (Fig. 60b) show?

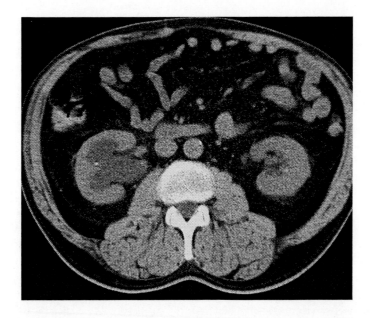

Fig. 60a

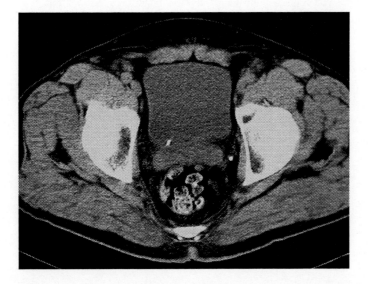

Fig. 60b

Answer 60: Obstruction of the right kidney secondary to a vesico-ureteric calculus

Findings: The right kidney demonstrates dilatation of the pelvicalyceal system. There is slight stranding in the perinephric fat. These changes are in keeping with obstruction. There is a tiny high-density lesion in a right calyx in keeping with a stone.

The CT section through the bladder demonstrates a calculus (arrow, Fig. 60c) at the right vesico-ureteric junction (VUJ) that was the cause of the obstruction.

CT has become the gold standard for identification of renal and ureteric stones and can demonstrate stones that are too small to identify on either ultrasound or intravenous urogram (IVU). It can also demonstrate renal tract obstruction and thus is useful for the investigation of renal colic and may incidentally demonstrate other renal and non-renal causes of acute abdominal pain.

Patients are scanned in the prone position with a full bladder. Prone scanning is performed to allow free intravesical stones to fall to the anterior aspect of the bladder so that they may be distinguished from stones in the VUJ. Scanning is performed from the kidneys to the bladder base. Oral and IV contrast media are not used in order to avoid masking stones. The majority of calculi (including radiolucent stones on plain film) appear as focal hyperdensities on CT. However, matrix and indinavir stones may be missed by CT as they are lucent due to their gelatinous composition. The secondary signs of calculi are: the ureteric rim sign (thickened ureter due to inflammation); hydronephrosis; hydroureter; renal enlargement; reduction in renal parenchymal density; delayed renal enhancement reflecting oedema; and also perinephric inflammatory stranding. Pelvic ureteric stones must be distinguished from phleboliths. The radiation dose using a low dose multidetector CT is just slightly higher than that of a three film IVU. However, CT IVU is still not in widespread use in UK hospitals because of the impact on the already overstretched CT service, extra cost implications, manpower considerations, and the increased radiation dose.

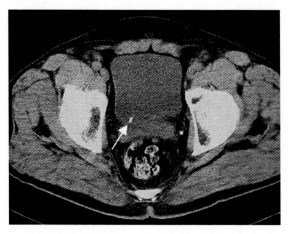

Fig. 60c   Pelvic CT section showing a right vesico-ureteric junction (VUJ) calculus (arrow).

Question 61

This 28-year-old man fell on an outstretched hand. What injury has he sustained (Fig. 61)?

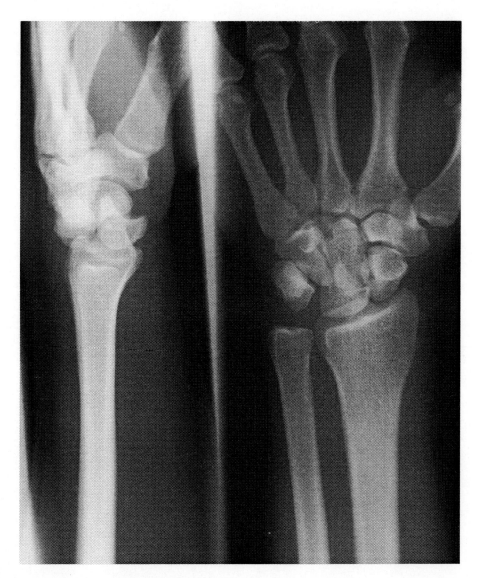

Fig. 61

Answer 61: Perilunate dislocation

Findings: On the lateral view there is dorsal dislocation of the distal carpal row due to disruption of the capitate–lunate joint. The lunate bone articulates normally with the radius although there is some rotation, giving it a triangular appearance on the anteroposterior (AP) film.

Carpal instability may be classified as follows:

Stage I   scapholunate ligament rupture with rotatory subluxation of the scaphoid. This is seen as the 'Terry Thomas' sign (widening of the scapholunate space that was likened to the gap between the upper incisors in the actor Terry Thomas) on the AP film;

Stage II   perilunate dislocation (as described in 'Findings');

Stage III   ligamentous disruption of the triquetrolunate joint due to injury of the radio-triquetral ligament and dorsal radiocarpal ligaments. This may be accompanied by triquetral malrotation, triquetrolunate dislocation, or triquetral fracture;

Stage IV   disruption of the radiolunate ligaments, which allows the lunate to become volarly displaced (lunate dislocation). This type of injury is commonly associated with a trans-scaphoid fracture.

Increasing severity of injury is seen from stage I to IV.

Question 62

This 56-year-old diabetic presented with right leg claudication. A distal aortogram is shown (Fig. 62a). What abnormality is shown? What management options are available?

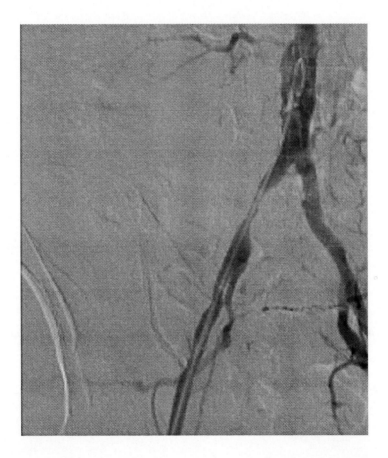

Fig. 62a

Answer 62: Severe stenosis of the right common iliac artery

Management options include percutaneous transluminal angioplasty (PTA), intravascular stent placement, and surgical aortofemoral grafting.

Factors that predict a favourable outcome from angioplasty:

- stenoses rather than occlusions, since in the latter condition it may not be possible to traverse the lesion with a guidewire;
- short (< 5 cm) concentric, smooth stenoses do better than long eccentric (irregular) lesions.

Indications for iliac artery stenting:

- a high residual aortoiliac systolic gradient (> 15 mmHg) after PTA;
- residual or recurrent stenosis (> 30%) after PTA;
- flow-limiting dissection at the angioplasty site;
- eccentric calcified stenoses fare better with stenting;
- iliac artery occlusions as there is a high risk of distal embolization and/or residual stenosis with PTA.

The 5-year patency rate of a common iliac PTA alone is approximately 70–75% compared with that of combined PTA and intravascular stenting, which is 90–95%. Common iliac artery lesions fare better than external iliac stenoses. In clinical practice PTA may be attempted initially, followed by stent deployment if a satisfactory angiographic result is not obtained (Figs 62b and 62c).

Aortobifemoral graft surgery is generally reserved for patients with extensive atheromatous disease and low surgical risk.

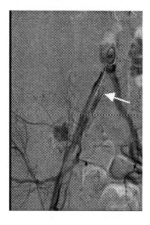

Fig. 62b   Percutaneous transluminal angioplasty (PTA) in this patient resulted in a flow-limiting dissection (arrow).

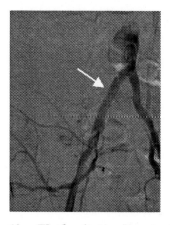

Fig. 62c   The flow-limiting dissection in Fig. 62b was successfully managed with a stent (arrow).

Question 63

This 45-year-old man presented with a 6-hour history of right loin pain. What does this renal ultrasound (Fig. 63) show and what is the diagnosis?

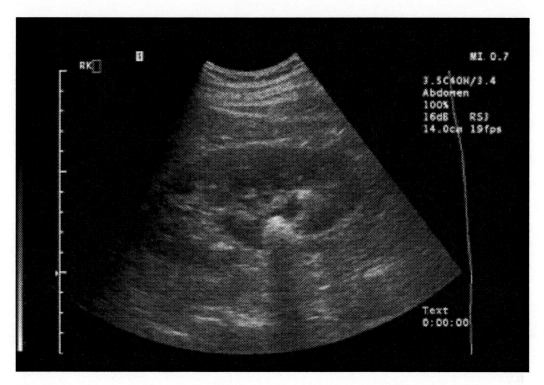

Fig. 63

Answer 63: Obstruction of the right kidney secondary to a calculus in the renal pelvis

Findings: There is right pelvicalyceal (PC) dilatation due to an obstructing calculus (seen as a bright oval lesion with posterior acoustic shadowing).

Ultrasound (US) is the modality of choice in the initial investigation of obstruction and often demonstrates the cause. US is able to demonstrate calculi and tumours of the renal pelvis, bladder, prostate, and pelvis as well as retroperitoneal pathologies. Ultrasound is a very sensitive detector of PC dilatation, the hallmark of obstruction. False-negatives occur due to the absence of PC dilatation, e.g. in early obstruction and in dehydrated states. Conversely, if the policy that PC dilatation equates with obstruction is adopted, a false-positive rate of up to 20% can be expected as there are several causes of non-obstructive PC dilatation—baggy renal pelvis, congenital megacalyces, secondary to a full bladder, post-obstructive dilatation, reflux, pregnancy, and overhydration. The most common of these causes is a 'baggy' renal pelvis (i.e. a slightly dilated non-obstructed pelvis), which can be easily diagnosed by US, IVU, or CT and obstruction excluded as there is no calyceal dilatation or functional evidence of obstruction. Furthermore, the degree of PC dilatation does not equate with the level of obstruction; the duration and degree of obstruction being more important factors. Colour Doppler ultrasound is useful in demonstrating the bilateral ureteric 'jets' of urine into the bladder, the presence of which excludes complete obstruction proximal to the vesico-ureteric junction.

Ultrasound may be unable to exclude obstruction in some situations, e.g. due to technical reasons (obese patients, small irregular echogenic kidneys), in renal cystic disease, in cases where large stones fill and distend the renal pelvis, in failure of dilatation of an obstructed system in severe parenchymal disease (acute tubular necrosis), in early obstruction, and in infiltrative processes such as retroperitoneal fibrosis. Under these circumstances further investigation is necessary. This may involve antegrade pyelography as part of a nephrostomy, radionuclide studies, high-dose urography, or CT. Percutaneous nephrostomy is indicated in obstruction in the presence of a pyonephrosis, severe loin pain, and in order to preserve renal function.

Question 64

This 33 year-old man developed chest pain and severe dyspnoea after a road traffic accident. The chest radiograph (Fig. 64) is shown. What is the diagnosis? What immediate action should be taken?

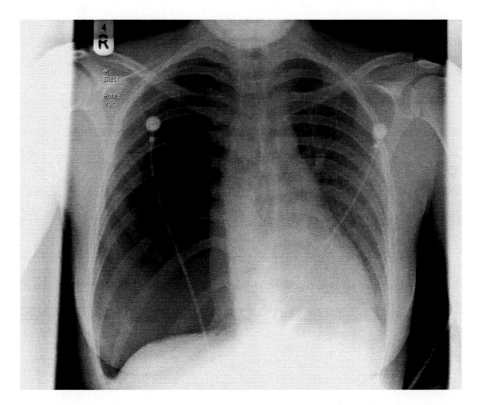

Fig. 64

Answer 64: Right tension pneumothorax

A tension pneumothorax is a medical emergency requiring immediate insertion of a venflon followed by a chest drain with underwater seal.

Findings: There is a right pneumothorax with mediastinal shift to the left. This radiograph should be unnecessary as the condition should be diagnosed clinically.

Tension pneumothorax is caused by a valvular mechanism occurring following a pneumo-thorax, resulting in air being sucked in during inspiration and not expelled during expiration, leading to positive intrapleural pressure. This causes mediastinal shift with compromise of venous return and cardiac output. A tension pneumothorax may be spontaneous or traumatic in aetiology.

A non-tension pneumothorax may be spontaneous, traumatic, or secondary to chronic obstructive pulmonary disease (COPD). Other causes include asthma, carcinoma, infections (e.g. pneumocystis carinii), lung abscess, pleural metastases, and interstitial lung disease.

Management may be conservative, with aspiration, chest tube drainage, or pleurodesis (± bleb resection).

Question 65

This 36-year-old man had a long history of upper abdominal pain. What is the high-density lesion (arrow) on this abdominal CT (Fig. 65) and where is it located? What condition does this patient have? What would be the most common cause in a child in the 'developed world'?

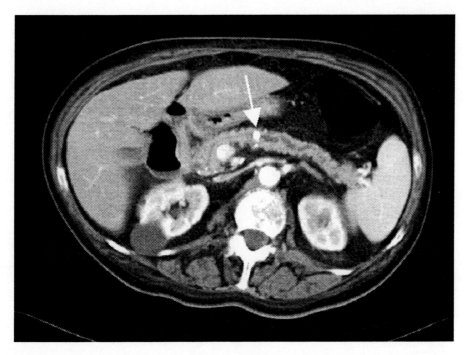

Fig. 65

Answer 65: A stone in a dilated main pancreatic duct

Chronic pancreatitis

Cystic fibrosis

Findings: The pancreas is atrophic in keeping with chronic pancreatitis. The main pancreatic duct is dilated distal to an obstructing stone.

Patients with chronic pancreatitis commonly present with a history of intermittent, acute epigastric pain that subsides (after about 7 years) with progressive destruction of the pancreas. Patients may also have jaundice from common bile duct obstruction (40%), steatorrhoea (80%), and diabetes mellitus (60%). Chronic alcohol abuse is the most common cause in adults.

In these patients, a chronic inflammatory process results in irreversible damage to the pancreas with protein plugs and calculi forming in the ducts of the gland.

The plain abdominal X-ray may show numerous irregular calcifications at the site of the pancreas (up to 50% of patients with alcoholic pancreatitis).

CT, ultrasound, ERCP, and MR all demonstrate chronic pancreatitis well. The main pancreatic duct is dilated (up to 70%) and commonly irregular (75%). The gland commonly is atrophic; with an irregular contour and up to three-quarters of patients show intraductal calculi. Areas of focal or even diffuse pancreatic enlargement can be seen at stages of the disease and the differential diagnosis from malignancy may be difficult. Other findings include: pseudocysts (30%), portal hypertension, arterial pseudoaneurysm formation, and thrombosis of the portal, mesenteric, and splenic veins.

Chronic pancreatitis is complicated by carcinoma of the pancreas in up to 4%.

Treatment is usually conservative, supportive, and symptomatic. However, infected pseudocysts commonly need drainage, and bile duct obstruction and bleeding from varices may require intervention.

Question 66

This neonate started vomiting 6 hours after birth. What does the abdominal radiograph (Fig. 66) show? Give two associated anomalies.

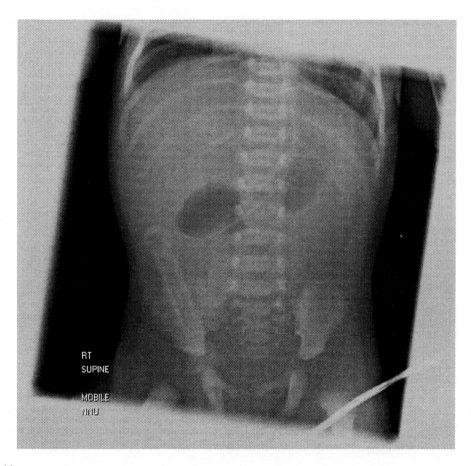

Fig. 66

Answer 66: Duodenal atresia

Associated anomalies include:

- Down syndrome (20–30%);
- gastrointestinal anomalies—oesophageal atresia, imperforate anus, biliary atresia, malrotation, duodenal duplication;
- congenital heart disease;
- renal anomalies;
- vertebral anomalies.

Findings: The stomach and duodenum are dilated giving the classic 'double bubble' sign of duodenal atresia. The rest of the abdomen is gasless. There is a nasogastric tube *in situ*.

Duodenal atresia is the most common cause of congenital small bowel obstruction. The 'double bubble sign' may also be seen in annular pancreas, duodenal web, duodenal stenosis, and obstruction due to duplication. The diagnosis is usually made on the plain abdominal radiograph without the need to perform contrast studies, which carry the risk of gastro-oesophageal reflux and aspiration.

Question 67

This 35-year-old lady presented with a cerebrovascular accident and an ischaemic left arm. The arch aortogram (Fig. 67) is shown. What is the diagnosis?

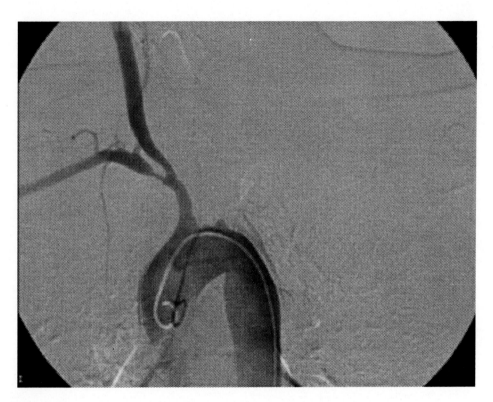

Fig. 67

Answer 67: Takayasu's arteritis

Findings: The left common carotid and subclavian arteries are completely occluded. Dimples of contrast are seen at their origins. There is a severe stenosis at the origin of the right subclavian artery.

Takayasu's arteritis (pulseless disease) is a large vessel vasculitis characterized by inflammation and fibrosis of the aorta and its main branches and the pulmonary arteries. It occurs in young Asian females (male:female 1:8), typically manifesting before the age of 30 years. It is characterized by two stages. Stage I (prepulseless phase) is the systemic phase of a few months duration with fevers, weight loss, arthalgia, and myalgia followed by stage II (pulseless phase), which consists of fibrotic changes leading to vessel stenosis and aneurysmal formation. This stage is characterized by hypertension, stroke, myocardial infarction, and limb ischaemia. The erythrocyte sedimentation rate (ESR) is elevated. Angiography typically shows long and diffuse/short and segmental irregular stenoses/occlusion of major branches of the aorta near their origins. Stenotic lesions of the thoracic aorta are more common than those of the abdominal aorta. Fusiform aortic aneuryms occur in 10–15%. Frequent skip areas are also a feature. It is the only form of aortitis that produces both stenosis and occlusion. Management consists of steroids, as well as surgical and angioplastic revascularization of stenotic lesions after resolution of active inflammation.

Question 68

This 69-year-old lady presented with vague abdominal pain and a change in bowel habit. A barium enema (Fig. 68a) and an unenhanced CT of the abdomen (Fig. 68b) were performed. What abnormality is present? What is the diagnosis? Is surgery indicated?

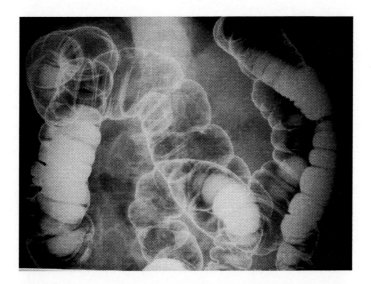

Fig. 68a

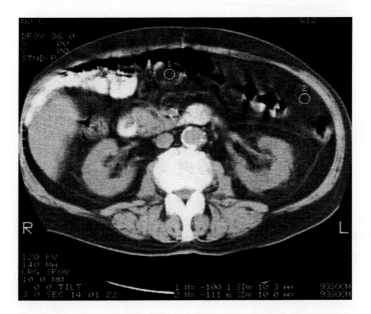

Fig. 68b

Answer 68: Colonic lipoma

Findings: The plain film (Fig. 68a) shows a well-defined lesion in the proximal transverse colon that is of reduced radiolucent density suggestive of a fatty composition. The mucosal over the lesion is smooth, consistent with a submucosal mass. The CT shows a well-defined mass. A region of interest (ROI) was been placed over the lesion (area 1) and its Hounsfield number (i.e. its quantitative density) is −100 HU consistent with fat. For comparison an ROI (area 2) has been measured at −111 HU in the adjacent mesenteric fat. See the section 'Computed tomography (CT)' in the introductory chapter for an explanation of the derivation of quantitative density.

Colonic lipomas are benign and therefore resection is unnecessary

Lipomas are the most common submucosal tumours of the colon. Colon lipomas are incidental findings and are usually asymptomatic but rarely may cause pain, haemorrhage, obstruction, or intussusception. Intestinal lipomas do not undergo sarcomatous transformation.

Question 69

What abnormalities are present on the barium enema (Fig. 69)? What is the diagnosis?

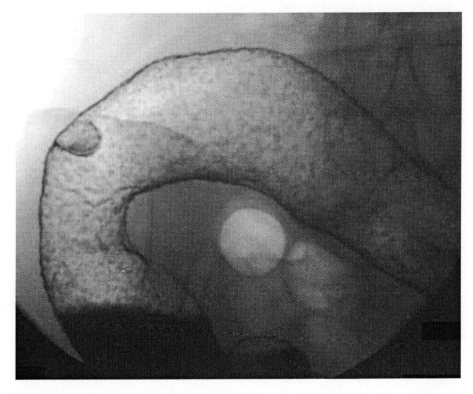

Fig. 69

Answer 69: Ulcerative colitis (UC) complicated by a carcinoma

Findings: There is 3 cm polypoid mass in the hepatic flexure. The mucosa of the colon is diffusely abnormal with a granular pattern consistent with superficial ulceration. There are no deep ulcers to suggest transmural disease. The colon is featureless with loss of the normal haustral pattern.

The incidence of colon cancer in ulcerative colitis ranges between 5 and 13% with a 25-fold increased risk after 7–8 years of UC. The risk of cancer is increased in pancolitis, in early onset of disease, and in primary sclerosing cholangitis. The most common sites of colon carcinoma in UC are the rectum and the descending and transverse colon. Therefore, UC patients require colonic surveillance to detect dysplastic change, which carries an increased risk of future cancer. In the presence of severe dysplasia elective colectomy may be performed.

Question 70

A 53-year-old man presented with deterioration in his conscious level. Precontrast (Fig. 70a) and postcontrast (Fig. 70b) CT brain scans were performed. What abnormalities are present? What is the most likely diagnosis?

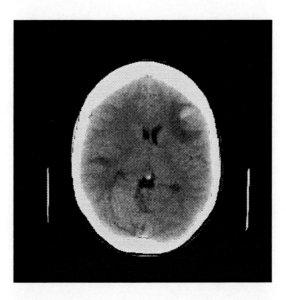

Fig. 70a

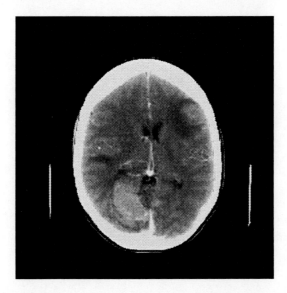

Fig. 70b

Answer 70: Haemorrhagic cerebral metastases

Findings: The precontrast image shows two hyperdense lesions in the left frontoparietal and right occipital lobes. The left frontoparietal lesion contains a high-attenuation anterior crescent-shaped area consistent with haemorrhage into a metastasis. Both lesions show vasogenic oedema of the adjacent white matter. Following intravenous contrast there is avid enhancement of the right occipital lesion and, to a lesser extent, of the left frontoparietal metastasis. The patient had a past history of melanoma. The CT brain appearances are consistent with metastatic melanoma.

Haemorrhagic metastases account for less than 5% of deposits and are most commonly from melanoma, oat cell lung carcinoma, renal cell carcinoma, choriocarcinoma, and thyroid carcinoma.

MRI is more sensitive than CT in the detection of cerebral metastases but the lesion characteristics are similar on the two modalities. Metastases are usually solid, with surrounding (vasogenic) oedema, and enhance strongly. Ring enhancement may be seen, which is also a feature of cerebral abscesses. However, abscesses may be differentiated from metastases by their central fluid density.

Metastases account for approximately 30% of intracranial tumours. The majority of lesions are supratentorial.

Five primary tumours account for 95% of metastases:

1   bronchial (50%, rarely squamous);
2   breast (15%);
3   gastrointestinal (15%);
4   renal cell carcinoma (10%);
5   melanoma (10%).

Calcified cerebral metastases occur in:

1   squamous cell carcinoma of the bronchus;
2   bone/cartilage-forming tumours;
3   mucinous adenocarcinomas (colon, ovary, pancreas, stomach);
4   thyroid (papillary);
5   testicular (teratoma);
6   post-radio/chemotherapy.

Cystic cerebral metastases occur in:

1   adenocarcinoma (bronchus, colon, ovary, pancreas, stomach);
2   squamous cell carcinoma of the bronchus.

Question 71

A 76-year-old lady developed fever and abdominal pain 5 days after an uneventful hysterectomy. What does the abdominal radiograph (Fig. 71a) show?

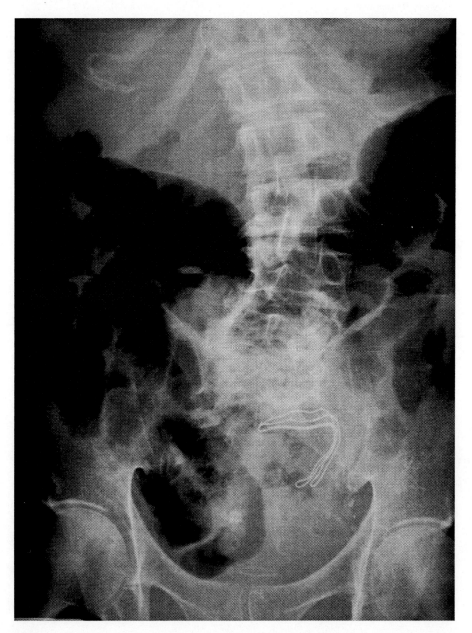

Fig. 71a

Answer 71: Retained surgical swab

Findings: There is a retained surgical swab in the pelvis. There are dilated small and large bowel loops consistent with an ileus.

A retained surgical swab acts as a nidus for infection with abscess formation, adhesions, bowel obstruction, and fistulae all possible sequelae. A retained surgical swab is recognized on radiographs or CT scans (Fig. 71b) by the radiodense stripe down the centre of the gauze.

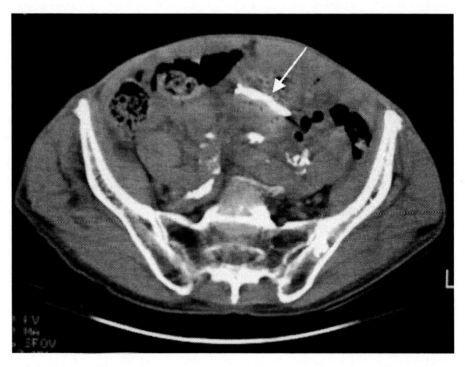

Fig. 71b   CT of the pelvis showing a retained swab (arrow).

Question 72

This 54-year-old man from southern China complained of gradually worsening nasal discharge. Describe the CT neck (Fig. 72a) findings. What is the most likely diagnosis? How is this condition best treated?

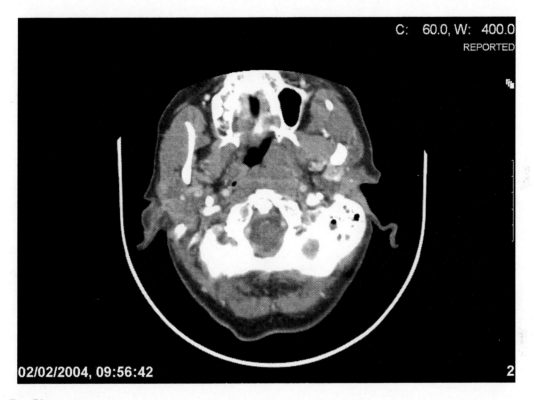

Fig. 72a

Answer 72: Nasopharyngeal carcinoma

Findings: There is asymmetry of the nasopharynx caused by a soft tissue mass (arrow, Fig. 72b) on the left arising posterolaterally, but extending across the midline posteriorly. It compresses the parapharyngeal space, and reaches the carotid sheath posterolaterally on the left and the pterygoid plates anteriorly on the left. The lateral pharyngeal recesses (fossae of Rosenmüller) and eustachian tube orifices are compressed.

This diagnosis of nasopharyngeal carcinoma is reached on the basis of the location of the tumour and the geographic origin of the patient but requires histological confirmation.

Nasopharyngeal carcinoma responds well to treatment with radiotherapy.

Nasopharyngeal carcinoma arises from squamous epithelial cells in the postnasal space. All the tumour cells carry the Epstein–Barr virus genome. Although it is a rare tumour world-wide, it has a high incidence in certain parts of the world and in certain races, such as south-east Asia, parts of north and east Africa, and in races living around the Arctic region (e.g. Inuits).

Presenting symptoms are usually due to local effects caused by the direct spread of the primary tumour mass, and therefore presentation is often late when extensive local invasion and lymph node metastases have already occurred. The tumour can spread extensively to involve the nasal and buccal cavities, oropharynx, paranasal sinuses, eustachian tubes, orbits and associated cranial nerves, skull base, lower cranial nerves (IX, X, XI, XII), and the parotid glands. Thus symptoms can include nasal blockage or discharge, deafness and middle ear disease, and ocular paresis. An unsuspected primary tumour may present with a lump in the neck or supraclavicular fossa from lymphatic spread to draining lymph nodes.

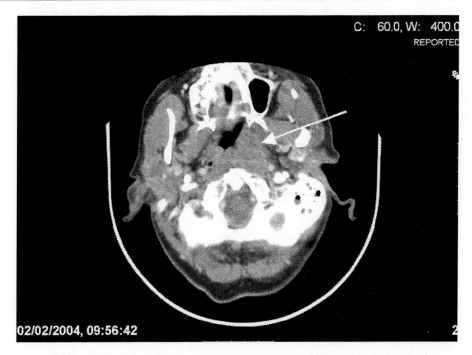

Fig. 72b   CT of the neck showing asymmetry of the nasopharynx caused by a soft tissue mass (arrow) on the left arising posterolaterally but extending across the midline posteriorly. Appearances are consistent with a nasopharyngeal carcinoma which was confirmed histologically.

Question 73

What abnormality does this radiograph (Fig. 73) show? Name an association.

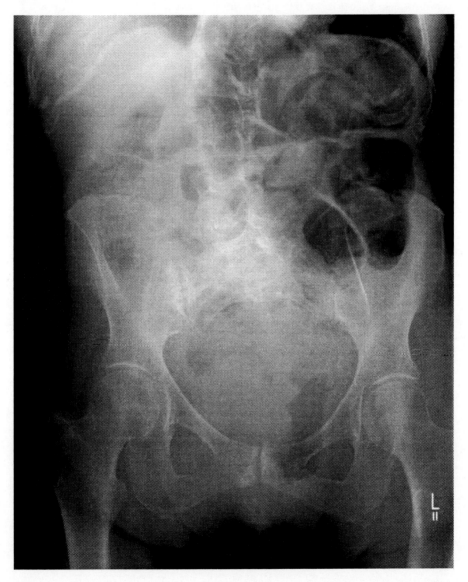

Fig. 73

Answer 73: Complete absence of the sacrum: sacral agenesis

The absence of the entire sacrum, rather than its destruction, makes this a congenital abnormality. There is also a scoliosis of the lumbar spine.

Associations include:

- musculoskeletal anomalies, especially of the legs (e.g. hip dislocation, ankle deformity);
- reduced bladder and bowel sphincter function/neurogenic bladder;
- spina bifida and its sequelae;
- maternal diabetes mellitus.

Question 74

This 72-year-old man complained of progressive leg weakness and numbness below his waist. What emergency condition does this sagittal T2-weighted MR (Fig. 74a) show? What should the immediate management be?

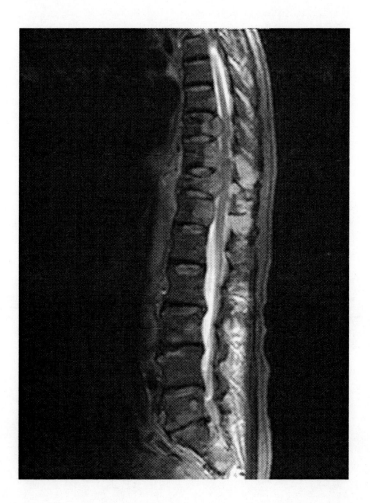

Fig. 74a

Answer 74: Spinal cord compression at the T9–T11 level due to metastatic carcinoma of the prostate

Findings: Metastases are seen as rounded lesions (of relatively high signal on these T2-weighted MR scans) in multiple vertebral bodies (Fig. 74a). The metastases in T9, T10, T11, and T12 are protruding from the posterior aspect of the vertebral bodies and their pedicles, and are severely narrowing the spinal canal compressing the cord. On the axial image through T9, the normally rounded spinal canal has been narrowed to a teardrop shape (arrow) by the encroaching metastases (arrowheads), and the CSF (white on these T2 images) is almost completely obliterated (Fig. 74b).

Urinary retention, if present, must be relieved by catheterization. Intravenous dexamethasone is given, and immediate radiotherapy administered to vertebrae at the level of acute cord compression. (The former to reduce cord oedema; the latter to shrink the metastases causing acute stenosis of the spinal canal, thereby trying to preserve neural function and prevent paraplegia.) In metastatic carcinoma of the prostate urgent bilateral subcapsular orchidectomy is indicated to eliminate stimulatory testosterone. Surgery more rapidly reduces plasma testosterone levels than chemical orchidectomy.

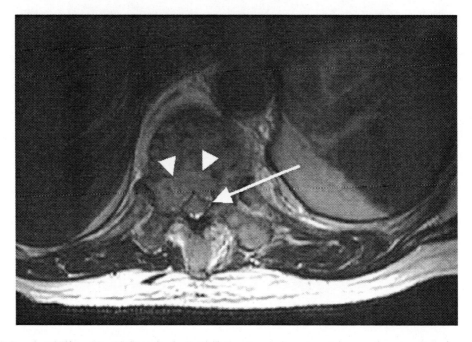

Fig. 74b   *Axial T2-weighted MR at the level of T9 showing cord compression secondary to vertebral metastases (arrowheads) narrowing the spinal canal (arrow).*

Question 75

This 21-year-old medical student sustained a twisting injury whilst playing squash. On examination his knee was painful and unstable. Describe the radiological abnormality on this sagittal T2-weighted MR (Fig. 75a). What is the diagnosis?

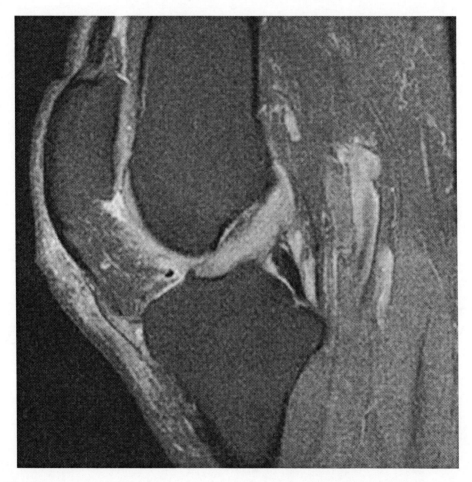

Fig. 75a

Answer 75: Partial rupture of the anterior cruciate ligament

Findings: The anterior cruciate ligament (ACL) is thickened with an irregular margin (arrow, Fig. 75b), and is of diffusely abnormal high signal. There is a joint effusion. Note the normal low signal posterior cruciate ligament (open arrow, Fig. 75b). The normal internal fibrillar structure of the cruciate ligament is lost, indicating that a significant number of its fibres have been torn, although some fibres of the ligament are still visible in continuity between its femoral and tibial attachments, so it is not completely disrupted. Also, there is no significant (> 5 mm) anterior subluxation of the tibia with respect to the femur, as would be expected were the ACL completely ruptured.

Up to 70% of ACL tears have associated medial meniscal and medial collateral ligament tears. Bone bruises (97%) are common in acute ACL injuries (although not seen on this particular image), and usually occur in the posterolateral tibial plateau, and in the midlateral femoral condyle, where bony impaction has taken place. It is important to diagnose partial tears of the ACL since these may progress to a complete tear and predispose to knee instability. Early surgical repair is indicated.

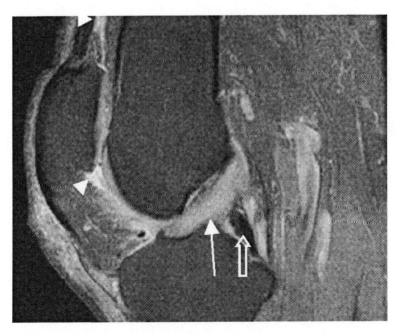

Fig. 75b   Sagittal T2-weighted MR of the knee showing a partial tear of the anterior cruciate ligament (arrow) and a joint effusion (arrowheads). Note the normal posterior cruciate ligament (open arrow).

Question 76

This is a gadolinium-enhanced axial T1-weighted image from an MR brain scan (Fig. 76) of a 24-year-old man with bilateral hearing loss. What is the diagnosis?

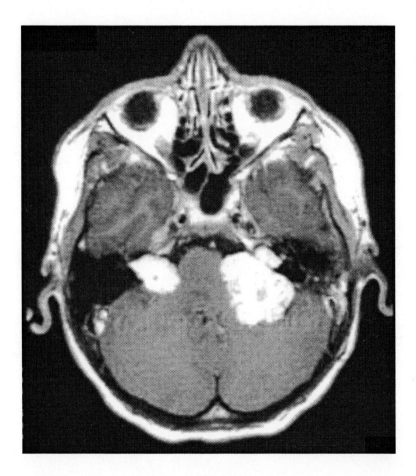

Fig. 76

Answer 76: Bilateral acoustic neuromas (Schwannomas)

Findings: There are bilateral intensely enhancing cerebellopontine angle (CPA) masses extending into the internal auditory canals. The lesions compress and distort the brainstem.

Bilateral acoustic neuromas are the hallmark of neurofibromatosis (NF) type 2. The tumour typically originates just within the internal auditory canal and grows into the CPA. Here it may compress the trigeminal and facial nerves and, less frequently, the glossopharyngeal and vagus nerves. As the tumour enlarges, the pons, lateral medulla, and cerebellum are compressed. Obstructive hydrocephalus may occur due to compression of the fourth ventricle. The most common early symptom is hearing loss with headache. Disturbed balance and gait are less common early symptoms.

NF type 2 is an autosomal dominant disorder, also associated with spinal meningiomas and cord ependymomas.

Imaging is central to the diagnosis of acoustic neuroma. CT may be used, but is not as sensitive as MRI, which will identify nearly all tumours.

The differential diagnosis for CPA masses is acoustic neuroma (75%), meningioma (10%), epidermoid (5%), and vascular lesions, metastases, and other primary intracranial tumours. The treatment of choice of acoustic neuroma is surgical excision. In most cases, the facial nerve can be preserved and in some cases the cochlear nerve as well.

Question 77

This 83-year-old lady was admitted with a history of 'being off her legs' for a few days. An abdominal radiograph (Fig. 77) was taken as part of her general investigation. What incidental abnormality is seen? What is the significance of this finding?

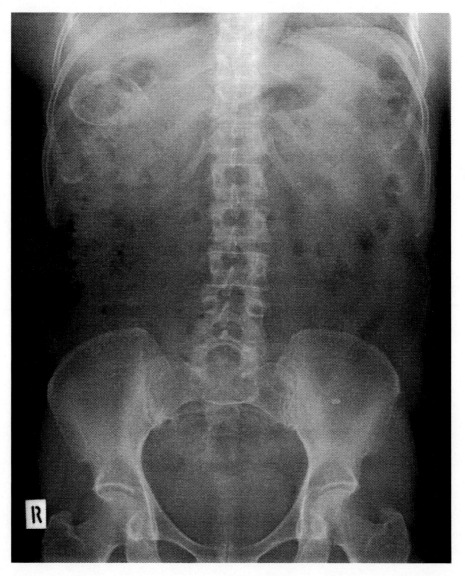

Fig. 77

Answer 77: Porcelain gallbladder

Findings: There is a rim of calcification around the gallbladder wall, known as 'porcelain gallbladder'. The differential diagnosis would be a calcified liver hydatid abscess/metastasis or a calcified renal lesion such as carcinoma or cyst.

Porcelain gallbladder is a precursor of carcinoma of the gallbladder in 10–20% of cases.

Porcelain gallbladder generally occurs in the elderly and is asymptomatic. It is associated with gallstones in the vast majority of cases (90%). It can affect part, or the whole, of the gallbladder wall. It may be diagnosed on a plain abdominal radiograph, or on CT (which is sensitive to smaller amounts of calcification), or on ultrasound where it is echogenic and casts a posterior acoustic shadow. Its malignant potential makes it an operable condition, if clinically appropriate.

Question 78

This 14-year-old complained of persistent pain in the right thigh for a month, and was now beginning to walk with a limp. Describe the radiological findings on the plain film (Fig. 78a). What is the diagnosis? What might an MR scan add to the assessment of the case?

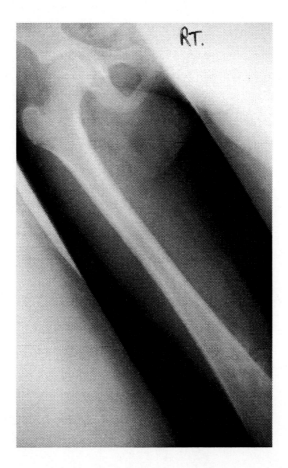

Fig. 78a

Answer 78: Osteosarcoma of the distal femur

Findings: There is an aggressive-looking lesion of the medial aspect of the distal femur, with new bone formation in a 'sun ray spiculation' pattern elevating the periosteum, giving a marked periosteal reaction ('Codman's triangle').

MR (Fig. 78b) shows the true extent of the bone marrow (open arrow) and soft tissue involvement (arrows). MR may also show intramedullary skip lesions, which occur in 25% of cases. MR is also useful for monitoring the response of patients undergoing chemotherapy, allowing the treatment regime to be changed if the response is poor. MR is sensitive in detecting local tumour recurrence. A bone scan and CT of the chest should also be performed as part of the staging process to look for distant metastases.

Osteosarcoma occurs with a prevalence of 5 in a million and comprises 20% of all primary malignant bone tumours. It most commonly affects adolescents aged 10–15 years, and occurs mainly in the metaphyses of long bones, especially the distal femur, proximal tibia, and humerus.

Preoperative chemotherapy is given for three reasons: to control micrometastases; to reduce the size of the primary tumour; and to reduce the peritumoral oedema. The surgery often requires amputation, although joint preservation is always attempted if the MR scan is favourable. The best prognostic indicator for survival is the degree of tissue tumour necrosis seen in the surgical specimen after the preoperative chemotherapy course—the greater the degree of necrosis, the better the chance of survival (91% survival with tumour necrosis > 90%; 14% survival with < 90% tumour necrosis).

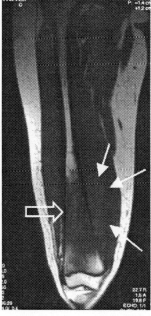

Fig. 78b   Coronal T1-weighted MR showing an osteosarcoma of the distal femur. MR demonstrates the full extent of the bone marrow involvement (open arrow) and soft tissue involvement (arrows) compared with the plain film.

Question 79

This 26-year-old man was involved in a road traffic accident. What abnormality is present on the lateral cervical spine radiograph (Fig. 79a)? How is this type of injury classified?

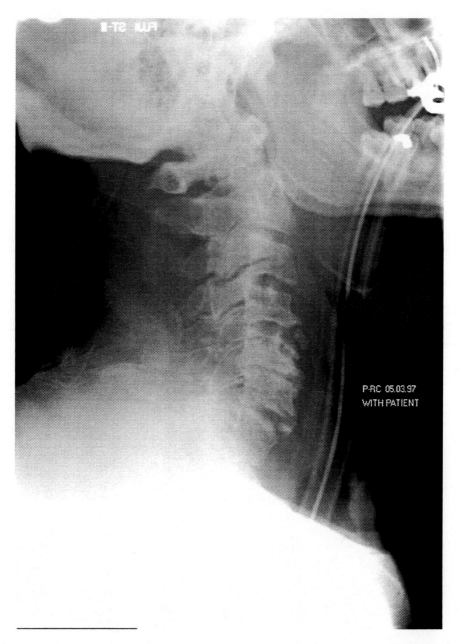

P-RC 05.03.97
WITH PATIENT

Fig. 79a

Answer 79: Fracture of the base of the odontoid peg (type II)

The classification of odontoid fractures is given in Table 1.

Findings: The C1 vertebra is displaced posteriorly with respect to the C2 vertebra. The fractured odontoid peg can be seen posterior to the anterior arch of C1. There is a sharp cut-off at the fracture site at the base of the odontoid peg. The patient is intubated indicating the severity of injury.

C2 fractures are common, accounting for 15–27% of cervical spine injuries. Fractures of the odontoid and neural arch account for 80% of C2 fractures. The mechanism of injury is hyperflexion. Odontoid fractures may be subtle and CT with reformatted images (Fig. 79b) is essential.

Table 1   Classification of odontoid fractures

Type	Incidence (%)	Complications
I (odontoid tip)	8	None
II (odontoid base)	59	Non-union (54–67%) Neurological symptoms (20%)
III (below odontoid)	33	Non-union (40%) if displaced more than 5 mm

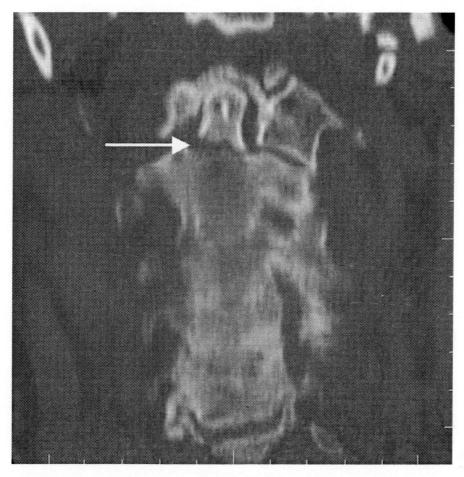

Fig. 79b   Coronal reformatted CT of the cervical spine showing a type II odontoid peg fracture (arrow).

Question 80

This Somalian refugee complained of difficulty in swallowing for the last 3 months and weight loss of 6 kg. What does the barium swallow (Fig. 80a) show? Give three differential diagnoses.

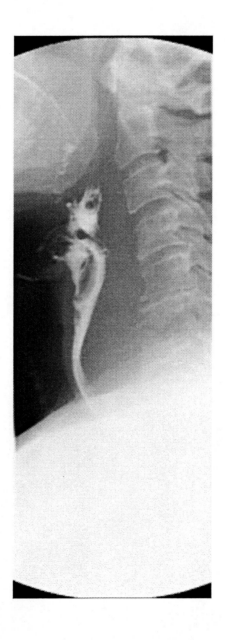

Fig. 80a

Answer 80: *Tuberculous prevertebral abscess associated with discitis*

Findings: The barium column is narrowed due to a smooth indentation on the posterior wall of the oesophagus. It is also deviated anteriorly by a midcervical soft tissue mass that is markedly widening the prevertebral space from C5 to C7. The oesophageal mucosal pattern is normal. Thus there is extrinsic compression of the upper oesophagus by a midcervical prevertebral mass. There is destruction of the inferior aspect of the C6 vertebral body and the superior part of the C7 vertebral body with loss of the disc space consistent with a discitis.

Possible diagnoses are:

- a prevertebral retropharyngeal cervical abscess. A tuberculous 'cold' paravertebral or prevertebral abscess is likely in this case because of the origin of the patient and the 3-month history. *Streptococcus pyogenes* is another common causative organism in retropharyngeal abscess;
- lymphadenopathy;
- an oesophageal duplication cyst;
- a posterior cervical tumour, e.g. neurofibroma;
- a retro-oesophageal thyroid goitre.

The CT of the neck (Fig 80b) confirms the presence of a prevertebral collection (A). It is of relatively low density (low attenuation) with some contrast enhancement posteriorly. This appearance is in keeping with pus within an abscess. There is marked patchy bony destruction of the adjacent vertebral body (arrows). The normal, avidly enhancing thyroid is seen anteriorly in front of the trachea (T). The oesophagus (arrowhead) is displaced anteriorly by the abscess, and is barely seen lying just behind the trachea.

It is highly likely that the infection started as a discitis that extended anteriorly. Tuberculous discitis usually starts in the anterior part of the intervertebral disc and spreads along the anterior spinal ligament to adjacent vertebrae, with progressive bony destruction. It is just possible that the mass could represent a necrotic mass of lymph nodes, but such extensive infiltrative bony destruction would be unlikely.

Narrowing of the oesophagus can be intrinsic (lesion arising within the lumen, such as a swallowed foreign body), intrinsic (arising within the wall), or extrinsic (compressing the oesophagus from outside). It is the prevertebral soft tissue mass, causing compression and anterior deviation of the oesophagus in this case, and the normal appearance of the oesophageal mucosa that indicate that there is extrinsic compression in this case.

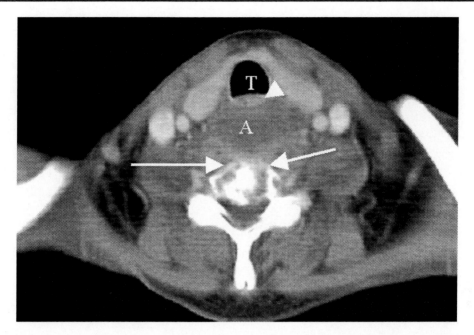

Fig. 80b   CT of the neck showing a prevertebral abscess (A) with destruction of the adjacent vertebral body (arrows). The oesophagus (arrowhead) is displaced anteriorly by the collection. T, Trachea.

Question 81

This 22-year-old student presented with recurrent nosebleeds. Her sister had chronic iron deficiency anaemia. What does this digital subtraction pulmonary arterial angiogram (Fig. 81) show? What is the underlying systemic condition, given the clinical history? How should lung lesions such as this be managed?

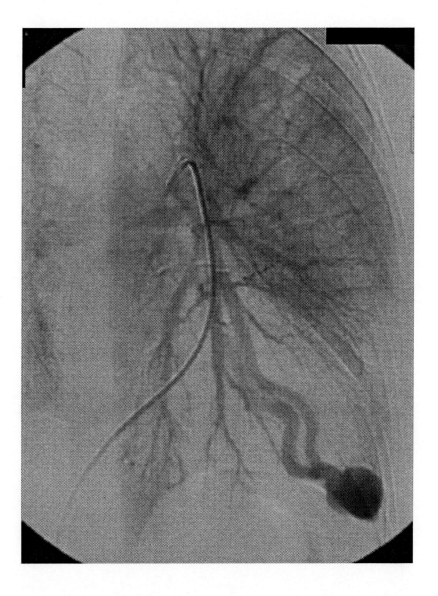

Fig. 81

Answer 81

Findings: A pulmonary arteriovenous malformation (PAVM), with a large feeding artery and early draining vein. The catheter is in the left main pulmonary artery.

Hereditary haemorrhagic telangiectasia (HHT) or Osler–Weber–Rendu syndrome

PAVMs that are large enough to cause significant shunting of deoxygenated blood through the lungs to the systemic circulation should be embolized (via a transvenous approach) using metallic coils (or small detachable balloons) to obliterate them.

HHT is a rare autosomal dominant condition where there are telangiectasiae of the mucous membranes (lips, mouth, nose, gastrointestinal and urinary tracts, skin) that can lead to recurrent epistaxes and occult gastrointestinal bleeding and chronic iron deficiency anaemia. Approximately a third of patients with a PAVM have HHT but only 15–20% of patients with HHT have PAVMs. The greatest risk of these PAVMs is cerebrovascular events due to paradoxical embolization through the right to left intrapulmonary shunts. These cerebrovascular complications include cerebral abscesses, strokes, or more minor transient ischaemic attacks. Embolization of PAVMs reduces the risk of these cerebrovascular events, and also reduces the right to left shunting thereby improving oxygen saturation, especially during exercise. Family members with HHT should be investigated by spiral CT scanning to identify possible PAVMs, which can be prophylactically embolized by interventional radiology.

Question 82

This patient presented with longstanding painless right ear discharge (otorrhoea) and, over the last few months, reduction of hearing in the right ear, which was found to be conductive on testing. Describe the abnormality on these thin CT coronal sections through the petrous temporal bones, on bony window settings (Figs 82a and 82b). What is the likely diagnosis, given the appearance of the lesion and the clinical history?

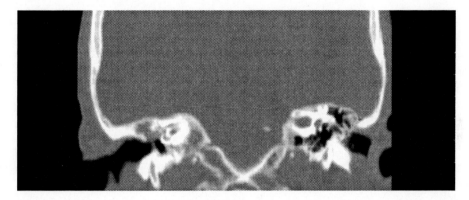

Fig. 82a

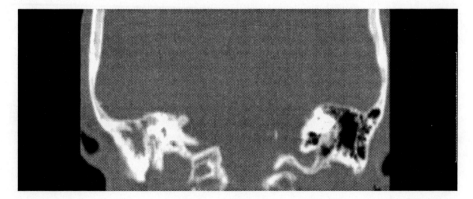

Fig. 82b

Answer 82: Cholesteatoma (epidermoid)

Findings: There is bony destruction of the epitympanum (arrowhead, Fig. 82c) (roof of the middle ear—the attic), which contains soft tissue (arrow, Fig. 82c). The scutum is eroded superiorly. The tegmen tympani (the roof of the epitympanum) is intact so the erosive process has not breached into the middle cranial fossa. The soft tissue (arrow, Fig. 82d) has extended via the aditus ad antrum to fill the air cells of the right mastoid.

Cholesteatoma is a squamous epithelial-lined sac filled with keratin debris leading to bone destruction by pressure and demineralizing enzymes. It is a destructive lesion of the temporal bone that gradually expands and causes complications by eroding adjacent bony structures. This can result in the destruction of the ossicles of the middle ear and otic capsule with hearing loss, vestibular dysfunction, facial paralysis, and intracranial complications.

The precise extent of bone erosion associated with cholesteatoma is well demonstrated by high-resolution thin-section CT of the petrous temporal bone in the coronal and axial planes. MR is better for demonstrating involvement of the meninges, veins and extension into the inner ear. Surgical planning generally requires both techniques to document destruction of thin bony structures and the relationship of the lesion to the dura and surrounding vessels.

The pathogenesis of cholesteatoma may be congenital or acquired (primary or secondary).

- Congenital cholesteatomas (epidermoid cysts) arise as a consequence of squamous epithelium trapped within the temporal bone during embryogenesis. They are most commonly found in the anterior mesotympanum or in the perieustachian tube area in early childhood (6 months to 5 years). Unlike other forms of cholesteatoma, congenital cholesteatomas are identified most commonly behind an intact and normal-looking tympanic membrane, without any history of recurrent suppurative ear disease, previous otological surgery, or tympanic membrane perforation.
- Primary acquired cholesteatomas (acquired epidermoids) arise as the result of tympanic membrane retraction. Local erosion can affect the lateral wall of the epitympanum (the scutum), the ossicles, and can proceed posteriorly through the aditus ad antrum into the mastoid, with exposure of the dura and/or erosion of the lateral semicircular canal with resultant deafness and vertigo.
- Secondary acquired cholesteatomas occur as a direct consequence of an injury to the tympanic membrane that can implant squamous epithelium into the middle ear—either a perforation from previous acute otitis media or trauma, or due to previous surgery to the drum.

The classical symptom of a cholesteatoma is painless otorrhea, either unremitting or frequently recurrent. Secondary infection of a cholesteatoma is very difficult to eradicate because the cholesteatoma has no blood supply, and so systemic antibiotics do not reach the centre of the cholesteatoma. Conductive hearing loss is also a common symptom of cholesteatomas, due to filling of the middle ear space with desquamated epithelium and/or to destruction of the ossicles. Tympanic membrane perforation is present in more than 90% of acquired cholesteatomas.

Surgical excision of the cholesteatoma is the only successful management.

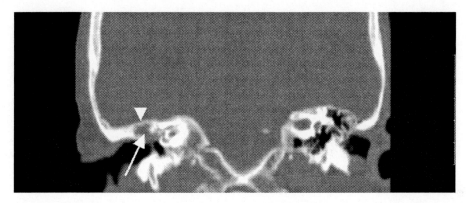

Fig. 82c   This thin CT section shows bony destruction of the epitympanum (roof of the middle ear—the attic, arrowhead), which contains soft tissue (arrow).

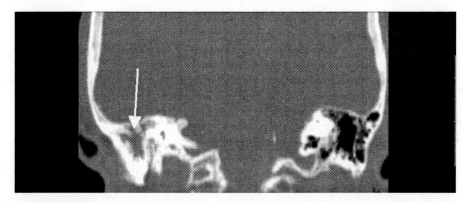

Fig. 82d   In this thin CT section the soft tissue (arrow) has extended via the aditus ad antrum to fill the air cells of the right mastoid.

Question 83

This 78-year-old man presented with weight loss and dysphagia. What two abnormalities does the CT section through the lower chest (Fig. 83a) show?

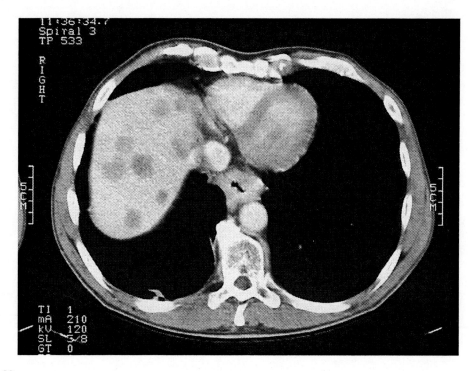

Fig. 83a

Answer 83: Carcinoma of the oesophageal with liver metastases

Findings: There are multiple focal hypodensities in the liver consistent with metastases (Fig. 83b). The distal oesophagus is thickened (arrow, Fig. 83b). Oesophageal carcinoma was proven on endoscopic biopsy.

Patients with carcinoma of the oesophagus present with dysphagia (90%, with duration of less than 6 months), weight loss (70%), retrosternal pain (50%), and regurgitation (30%).

Oesophageal carcinoma is relatively uncommon (< 1% of all cancers and 5% of gastro-intestinal malignancies). Predisposing factors include achalasia and caustic stricture (both 1000 × risk), Barrett's oesophagus, tobacco, asbestosis, and alcohol.

Histologically, tumour type is most commonly squamous cell (95%). Adenocarcinoma accounts for the majority of the remaining cases (it is the most common tumour type when carcinoma complicates Barrett's oesophagus). Less common tumour types include carcino-sarcoma, adenoid cystic carcinoma, and mucoepidermoid carcinoma.

The diagnosis may be confirmed by endoscopy or barium swallow. Barium swallow most commonly shows a polypoid/fungating lesion, but can show a large ulcer, gradual smooth narrowing, or varicoid form.

CT is useful for staging oesophageal carcinoma. Detection of a small, primary oesophageal neoplasm can be difficult, particularly at the gastro-oesophageal junction. When determining distant metastatic spread it is important to look for: displacement/compression of the airways (90+% accuracy for invasion); evidence of fistulation to the airways; contact with the aorta (> 90 degree arc suggests non-resectability); lymphadenopathy; and liver, lung, and adrenal metastases. Interventional radiology is useful in placing palliative stents.

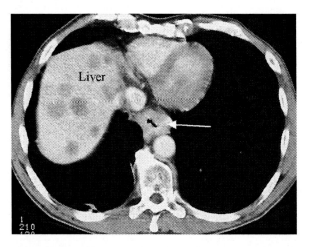

Fig. 83b CT through the lower chest showing multiple liver metastases and a thickened irregular distal oesophagus (arrow). Oesophageal carcinoma was proven on endoscopic biopsy.

Question 84

This 57-year-old cook complained of longstanding heartburn and a worsening sensation of food sticking after swallowing, especially lumps of meat. What does the barium swallow show (Fig. 84)? What would be the next investigation?

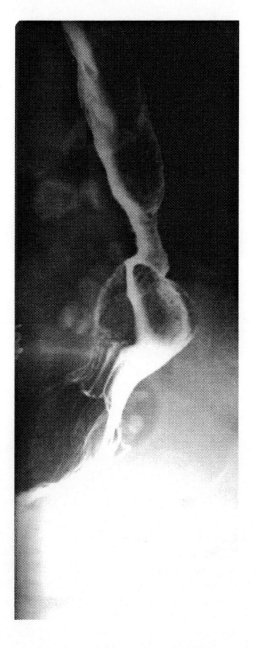

Fig. 84

Answer 84: Benign oesophageal stricture

Findings: The barium swallow shows a 4 cm smooth, circumferential, distal oesophageal stricture above a moderate-sized sliding hiatus hernia.

The next investigation should be a flexible oesphagoscopy with inspection and biopsy of the stricture. (Even though the stricture has smooth margins and therefore looks benign, direct visual inspection with biopsies is important to fully to exclude Barrett's oesophagus and malignancy.)

In adults, gastro-oesophageal reflux disease (GORD)-induced strictures of the lower oesophagus account for the majority of benign oesophageal strictures. In most patients with GORD the symptoms are well controlled by lifestyle changes, antacids, and proton pump inhibitor medication, and the oesophageal mucosa is not damaged. In the minority where mucosal ulceration develops, the inflammatory process spreads through the oesophageal wall. Stricture is the end result of ulceration and is due to granulation and scar contracture. Stricture usually only occurs after years of symptomatic reflux ('heartburn' and, sometimes, dysphagia). Depending upon severity, benign oesophageal strictures may be treated with dilatation—generally balloon dilatation performed under radiological fluoroscopic guidance, but also by direct vision endoscopic dilatation. This procedure generally needs to be repeated as the stricture recurs.

A hiatus hernia occurs when a portion of the stomach passes though the oesophageal hiatus between the crura of the diaphragm (at T10 level). There are two types of acquired non-traumatic hiatus hernias: sliding and paraoesophageal. The sliding hiatus hernia is the most common, and occurs when the lower oesophageal sphincter (LES), together with a portion of the adjacent stomach, moves into the chest. The paraoesophageal (or rolling) hiatus hernia occurs when the fundus of the stomach herniates into the chest through the oesophageal hiatus, but the gastro-oesophageal junction (and LES) remain below the diaphragm.

Factors predisposing to hiatus hernia are:

- causes of raised intraabdominal pressure, i.e. obesity, pregnancy, ascites, chronic straining at stool (possibly due to constipation from low fibre diets);
- increasing age: thought to be due to muscle weakening and loss of tissue elasticity.

Hiatus hernias are relatively common and the vast majority are asymptomatic. In a minority of people sliding hiatus hernias may worsen existing GORD. There are several mechanisms whereby this may occur. The hiatus hernia can act as a fluid trap increasing the time during which the gastric acid is in contact with the oesophageal mucosa. Also, when the LES is in the chest, it is less effective as a sphincter because its mechanics are altered, i.e. it is situated in a low pressure area in the chest, and it undergoes more frequent episodes of transient relaxation. The paraoesophageal (rolling) type of hiatus hernia does not exacerbate GORD, but is associated with volvulus and strangulation and so is often operated upon prophylactically.

Question 85

This 57-year-old man was brought to casualty in a coma following a head injury. What does the unenhanced CT of the brain (Fig. 85) show?

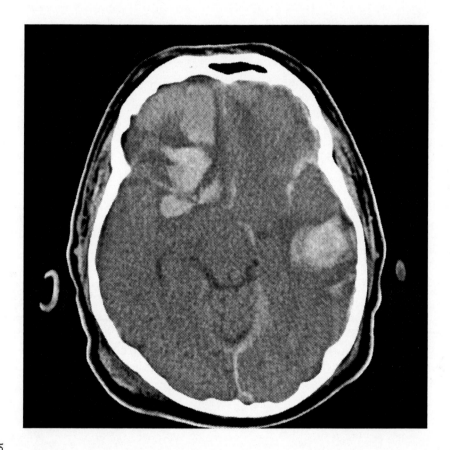

Fig. 85

Answer 85: Multifocal intracerebral haemorrhage

Findings: There are two large recent cerebral haemorrhages, one in the right frontoparietal region and another in the left temporoparietal region. There is fresh blood in the subarachnoid space as demonstrated in the left sylvian fissure, along the falx, and over the tentorium cerebelli. The haematomas are causing mass effect shown by the compression of the temporal horn of the left lateral ventricle and the suprasellar and ambient cisterns.

The aetiology of intracerebral haemorrhage includes:

- aneurysm (33%)
- hypertension (33%)—most often located in the basal ganglia or thalamus (75%), more commonly in the elderly;
- arteriovenous malformation (10%);
- trauma;
- haemorrhagic infarction;
- bleeding into tumour;
- coagulopathy.

The features of a cerebral haematoma on non-enhanced CT vary according to age. In the first 24 hours blood is seen as a homogeneous high-attenuation lesion with a well defined periphery. As the haematoma consolidates, layering is often seen and its attenuation decreases so that there is a stage between 3 and 10 weeks when it is isointense with surrounding brain and has an associated hypointense rim. During resolution, osmotic fluid uptake may cause the cerebral haematoma to appear hypointense compared with surrounding brain.

CT is superior to MR in the identification of acute haemorrhage as acute blood may be isointense to brain on MR. Mass effect of the haematoma or blood in the ventricles may obstruct the flow of cerebrospinal fluid (CSF) producing hydrocephalus.

Question 86

This 57-year-old lady presented to Accident and Emergency with sudden onset headache and photophobia. An unenhanced CT brain was performed (Fig. 86). What is the diagnosis?

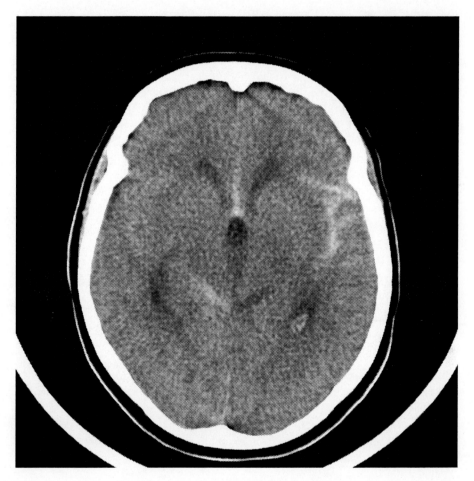

Fig. 86

Answer 86: *Subarachnoid haemorrhage*

Findings: The CT scan image demonstrates acute subarachnoid blood (white because of its higher density) in the ambient cistern, in the interhemispheric sulcus, and sylvian fissures.

Subarachnoid haemorrhage most frequently occurs due to ruptured aneurysm (72%) or arteriovenous malformation (10%). Less commonly, it is caused by hypertension, blood dyscrasias, tumours, and trauma causing bleeding usually from leptomeningeal vessels at the vertex.

Imaging is useful in identifying the cause and complications of subarachnoid haemorrhage. The accuracy of CT is approximately 90% in the first day after onset, decreasing thereafter, with persistence of blood after 4 days only in massive haemorrhage. Lumbar puncture is obligatory if the CT is normal since subarachnoid blood is not always visible on CT. MR is relatively insensitive acutely, but MR angiography is accurate in demonstrating the presence of circle of Willis aneurysms. Many still regard four-vessel angiography as the gold standard for identification of aneurysms. Twenty per cent of patients have multiple aneurysms. If multiple aneurysms are present, indicators as to which one has bled are: the largest aneurysm (> 5 mm); loculated aneurysm; anterior communicating artery aneurysms; adjacent vasospasm and haematoma.

The sites of symptomatic aneurysms angiographically are:

- posterior communicating artery, 38%;
- anterior communicating artery, 36%;
- middle cerebral artery (branching point), 21%;
- terminal internal carotid artery, 13%;
- basilar and posterior inferior cerebellar arteries, 3%.

Complications of subarachnoid haemorrhage are common and include obstructive hydrocephalus and vasospasm. Obstruction is caused in the early phase by blood obstructing the aqueduct of Sylvius, fourth ventricle, or, less commonly, the interventricular foramina of Munro. After 1 week or more a communicating hydrocephalus can develop due to damage to the arachnoid villi. Cerebral vasospasm most commonly occurs between 7 to 10 days after haemorrhage and may lead to ischaemia and infarction.

Question 87

This 51-year-old alcoholic presented 4 days after a head injury with confusion and a dilated right pupil. What does the unenhanced CT brain scan (Fig. 87) show?

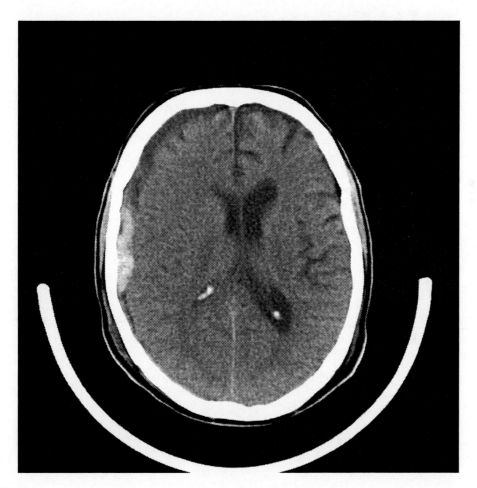

Fig. 87

Answer 87: Acute on chronic right subdural haematoma

Findings: There is a focal area of hyperdensity in the right subdural space bounded by a hypodense subdural collection consistent with an acute on chronic subdural haematoma. There is mass effect as demonstrated by the ipsilateral sulcal effacement and midline shift to the left.

Subdural haematomas are predominantly seen in infants and the elderly (the latter having a large subdural space due to cerebral atrophy). Predisposing factors are alcoholism, epilepsy, and coagulopathies. Damage to the 'bridging veins' that connect the cortical veins on the surface of the brain to the dural sinuses causes bleeding into the subdural space between the dura and arachnoid. This space does not extend into the sulci (unlike subarachnoid blood) and extends freely across sutural lines (whereas extradural blood is limited by sutural lines).

Subdural haeamtomas appear on CT as extra-axial collections with a concave inner border (unlike extradural haematomas, which have a convex inner border). They most commonly occur along the cerebral convexity but they can extend along the interhemispheric fissure and the tentorium.

The age of the subdural haematoma may be judged approximately from its appearance. If it is denser than brain (hyperdense) it is probably less than 1 week old. If it is the same density as brain (isodense) then it is probably 1–2 weeks old. This group can be difficult to diagnose. After 3–4 weeks the collection becomes hypodense compared with normal brain. The skull vault should be inspected for fractures, although studies have shown no consistent relationship between fractures and subdural haematomas (unlike extradural haematomas where skull fractures are generally associated). A large percentage of patients have no history of head injury.

Question 88

This 43-year-old man presented with worsening headaches and a bitemporal hemianopia on examination. A coronal contrast-enhanced MR through the pituitary fossa (Fig. 88a) is shown. Describe the radiological features. What is the diagnosis?

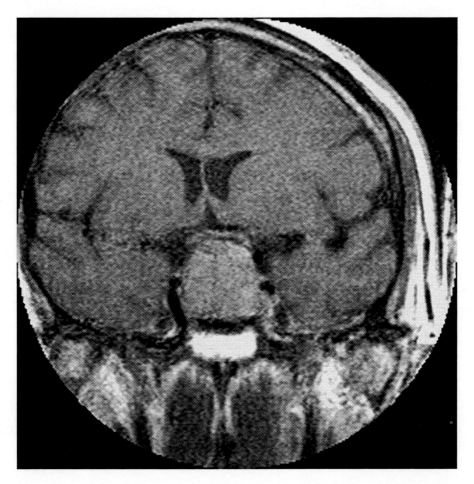

Fig. 88a

Answer 88: Pituitary macroadenoma

Findings: There is a large, slightly inhomogeneous mass (arrow) filling the sella turcica and extending upwards (note its convex upper border) displacing the optic chiasm superiorly (open arrow, Fig. 88b).

Pituitary adenomas may be divided into micro- (20–30%) and macroadenomas (70–80%) on the basis of size, 10 mm craniocaudal length being the cut-off. Both derive from the anterior pituitary gland. Macroadenomas are usually endocrinologically inactive and thus present with symptoms relating to their mass effect, such as headache (which may be due to hydrocephalus secondary to compression of the foramina of Monro), bitemporal hemianopia due to compression of the optic chiasm, and cranial nerve sinuses (III, IV and VI) involvement within the cavernous.

MR is the preferred method of investigation as it easily allows multiplanar imaging with coronal and sagittal planes being routinely used. Both micro- and macroadenomas are slightly lower in signal on T1 weighting and in 30–50% show higher signal on T2 weighting with respect to the normal pituitary gland (the latter finding is more common in macroadenomas). Microadenomas enhance less avidly than normal pituitary appearing relatively hypointense compared with the rest of the normal gland, whereas macroadenomas intensely enhance in an inhomogeneous manner. Note in this case that the upper border of the pituitary is convex upwards; a relatively reliable sign of a pituitary lesion. Other signs that may be present include erosion or depression of the floor of the sella, invasion of the cavernous sinuses, and thickening and/or displacement of the stalk.

Microadenomas tend to be endocrinologically active and thus present earlier. They are seen as small hypointense lesions on pre- and postcontrast-enhanced T1-weighted sequences. The most common type is the prolactinoma. Others include adenocorticotrophic hormone (ACTH)-, growth hormone (GH)-, follicle stimulating hormone/luteinizing hormone (FSH/LH)-, and thyroid stimulating hormone (TSH)-secreting tumours. They cannot be differentiated on imaging criteria.

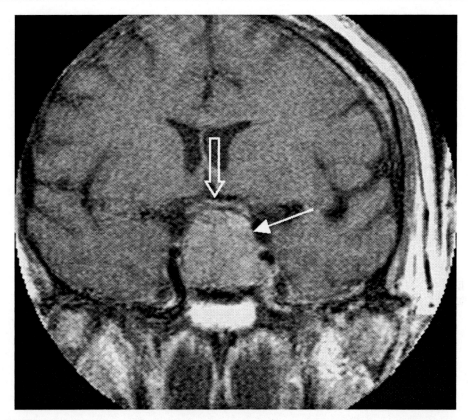

Fig. 88b   This coronal contrast-enhanced MR through the pituitary fossa shows a large, slightly inhomogeneous mass (arrow) filling the sella turcica and extending upwards displacing the optic chiasm superiorly (open arrow). Appearances are consistent with a pituitary macroadenoma.

Question 89

This 82-year-old lady complained of a rapidly increasing left-sided neck mass and difficulty in swallowing. Describe the abnormalities on the contrast-enhanced CT of the neck (Fig. 89a). What is the diagnosis?

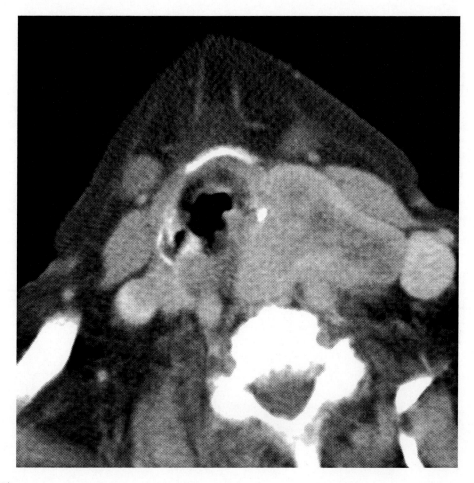

Fig. 89a

Answer 89: Thyroid carcinoma

Findings: The CT (Fig. 89b) demonstrates a large heterogeneous mass (arrow) arising from and replacing the left thyroid lobe, which has invaded the left thyroid cartilage. The left internal jugular vein is displaced laterally and the left common carotid artery posteriorly. Anaplastic thyroid carcinoma was found on fine needle aspiration.

Thyroid cancer is uncommon accounting for less than 1% of all malignant neoplasms. Less than 10% of all palpable thyroid nodules are malignant. However, benign nodular pathologies (most frequently nodular hyperplasia and adenomas) are common with a prevalence of 13–50% on ultrasound. The majority are impalpable.

Thyroid cancer is of four different histological types. The most common is papillary thyroid carcinoma, accounting for 60% and frequently seen in females in their forties. It is usually a well-differentiated tumour that spreads into regional lymph nodes.

On ultrasound papillary thyroid carcinoma is usually hypoechoic, hypervascular, and demonstrates microcalcifications due to calcified psammoma bodies. The prognosis is good with a 90% 10-year survival.

Follicular carcinomas account for 20% of thyroid carcinomas and again are seen most frequently in females in their forties. These tumours metastasize early to lung and bone. They are impossible to assess well by radiological means as their appearances are indistinguishable from those of benign follicular adenoma and even fine needle aspiration cytology is not helpful as vascular and capsular invasion are the only reliable signs of malignancy. Follicular carcinomas are frequently seen in thyroid glands with other adenomatous or hyperplastic nodules. There is a 70% 10-year survival.

Anaplastic thyroid carcinoma is the least common (10–15% of thyroid malignancies) and most aggressive, with early dissemination and invasion of local structures such as the larynx and vascular structures. The prognosis is poor with a 5% 5-year survival.

Medullary carcinoma of the thyroid is seen in association with type II multiple endocrine neoplasia.

CT is useful in staging thyroid carcinomas (local and distant spread) and in assessing retrosternal extension of goitres.

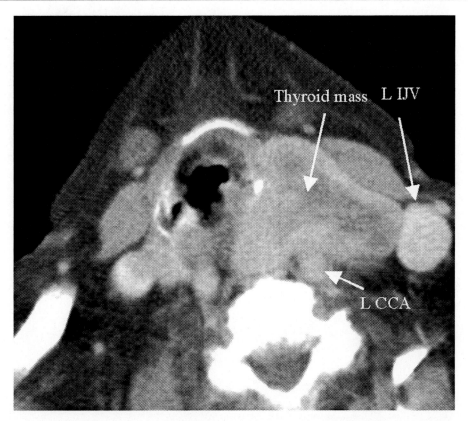

Fig. 89b CT of the neck showing a thyroid carcinoma arising from the left thyroid lobe and invading the left thyroid cartilage. The left internal jugular vein (L IJV) is displaced laterally and the left common carotid artery (L CCA) posteriorly.

Question 90

This 80-year-old lady was 1 week post internal fixation of a fractured neck of femur when she complained of acute dyspnoea. What does this contrast-enhanced CT of the chest (Fig. 90a) show?

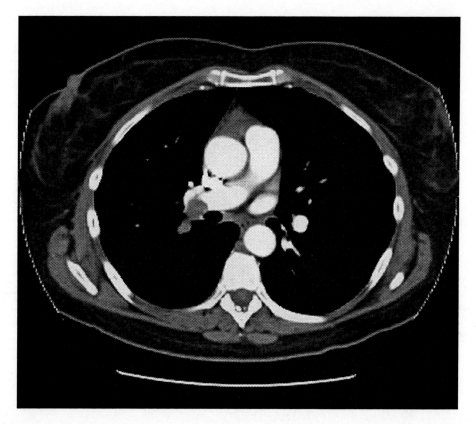

Fig. 90a

Answer 90: Pulmonary embolism (PE)

Findings: There is a filling defect in the right main pulmonary artery (arrow, Fig. 90b) also depicted on a coronal reformatted image (curved arrow, Fig. 90c) consistent with a large pulmonary embolus.

PE is a well-recognized complication of surgery especially knee and hip surgery. Other risks include age, immobility, smoking, the oral contraceptive pill, and previous deep vein thrombosis (DVT) or PE. The majority of pulmonary emboli arise from the deep veins of the leg (90%) and a smaller number from the deep veins of the pelvis. A much smaller number derive from implantable devices such as renal dialysis lines and caval filters. Only about 25% of all fatal PEs are symptomatic for DVT ante mortem.

The chest radiograph (CXR) is usually the first line of radiological investigation. There are a multitude of signs associated with PE including subsegmental atelectasis (small volumes of collapse seen as linear densities), consolidation, infarction, and pleural effusion. There are also some well-recognized signs including the Westermark sign (focal reduction in pulmonary blood flow due to PE) and the Fleischner sign (dilatation of the pulmonary artery proximal to an embolus). These signs are non-specific. Given the low sensitivity and specificity of CXR it is no longer useful for diagnosis but as a guide to the next most useful investigation. Those with a normal or near normal CXR should have a ventilation/perfusion (V/Q) scan (Fig. 90d) and those with an abnormal CXR should have a CT pulmonary angiogram (CTPA). The advantages of a V/Q scan are the lower radiation dose and no exposure to contrast. The difficulty with a V/Q scan is that any abnormality seen renders it 'intermediate' in probability for the presence of a PE. It must be remembered that a normal or low-risk V/Q scan has the same negative predictive value as a normal CTPA.

CTPA demonstrates PEs as intraluminal filling defects or as contrast surrounding the thrombus ('polo mint' sign). CTPA is equal to angiography in the sensitivity of detection of PEs down to the subsegmental level and, unlike pulmonary angiography, is a non-invasive investigation. CTPA is useful in the emergency situation when a V/Q scan will not be available. The sensitivity and specificity of CTPA in the detection of PE are 80% and 85%, respectively.

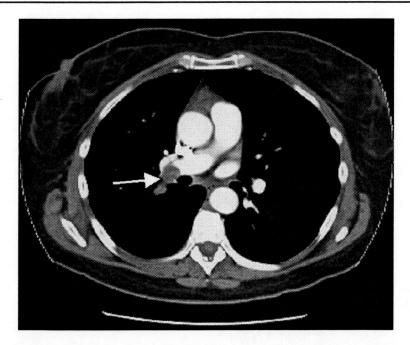

Fig. 90b   CT pulmonary angiogram showing a filling defect in the right main pulmonary artery (arrow) consistent with an embolus.

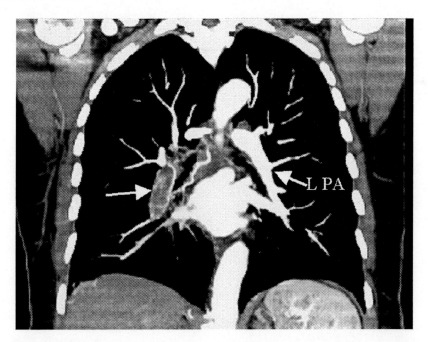

Fig. 90c   CT coronal reformatted image showing an embolus in the right pulmonary artery (arrow). Note the normal patent left pulmonary artery (L PA).

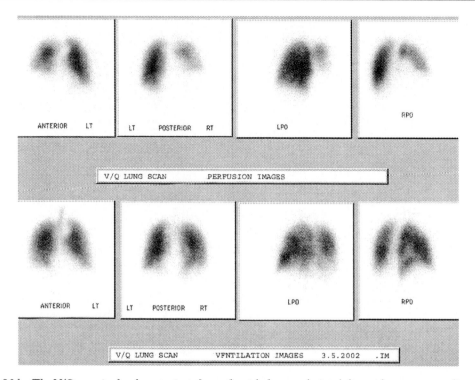

Fig. 90d *The V/Q scan in the above patient shows the right lung perfusion defect with no corresponding ventilation defect (mismatched defect) consistent with a PE.*

Question 91

This 62-year-old man who had undergone a rigid sigmoidoscopy for rectal bleeding complained of abdominal pain following the procedure. What abnormalities are present on this abdominal film (Fig. 91a)?

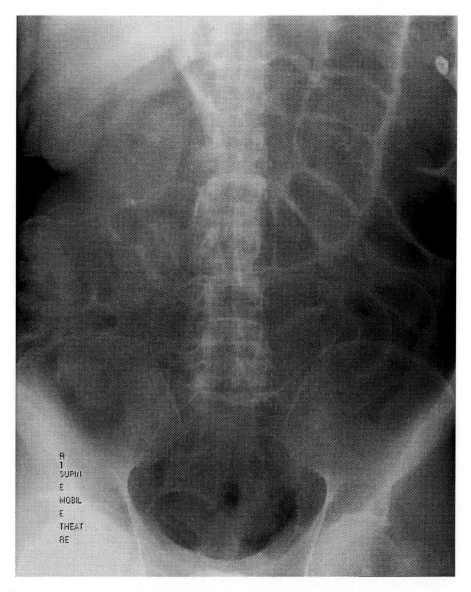

Fig. 91a

Answer 91: Pneumoperitoneum

Findings: There is free intraperitoneal gas (pneumoperitoneum) throughout the abdomen as shown by the presence of gas on either side of the large (arrows, Fig. 91b) and small bowel wall (Rigler's sign). The falciform ligament (open arrows, Fig. 91b) is also outlined by intraperitoneal gas. This was due to biopsy-induced perforation of the sigmoid colon.

Other signs of free intraperitoneal gas (not shown on this film) are:

- air outlining the umbilical ligament;
- air interposed between the colon and properitoneal fat stripe of the abdominal wall;
- a central collection of gas anterior to loops of bowel (football sign) on a supine patient;
- on an erect chest radiograph air collects under the hemidiaphragms. The erect chest radiograph is the best simple investigation for detecting intraperitoneal air. It is imperative that a delay of 5–10 minutes occurs from the patient being put in an upright position and the film being taken to allow the gas to rise. However, the gas may not rise if it is trapped by adhesions.

A left lateral decubitus film (patient lying on his/her left side) detects as little as 1 ml of free air. The patient remains in position for 5–10 minutes prior to taking the radiograph to allow any free air to rise. The edges of the liver will be seen in sharp relief against the abdominal wall if free gas is present. However, it is important to recognize the signs of free intraperitoneal gas on supine films as the patient may be too ill to obtain other films.

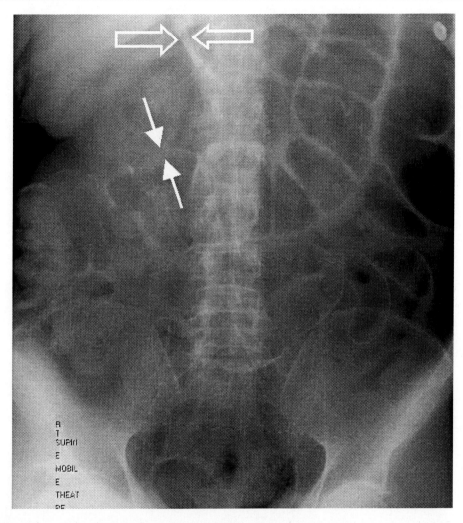

Fig. 91b   Abdominal radiograph showing free intraperitoneal gas (pneumoperitoneum) throughout the abdomen as shown by the presence of gas on either side of the large bowel wall (arrows; Rigler's sign). The falciform ligament (open arrows) is also outlined by intraperitoneal gas.

Question 92

This 42-year-old man complained of headaches. A contrast-enhanced CT of the brain was performed (Fig. 92). Describe the abnormality and suggest a diagnosis.

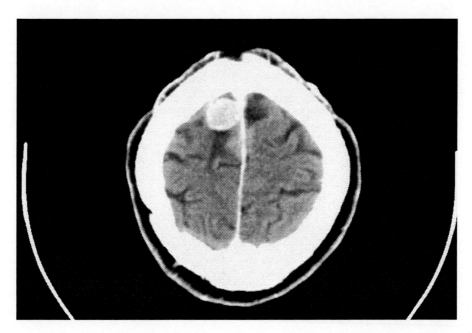

Fig. 92

Answer 92: Meningioma

Findings: There is a 2 cm well-defined homogeneously enhancing mass abutting the right side of the falx. There is no surrounding oedema. This tumour has the appearances of a meningioma.

Meningiomas are extraaxial benign tumours. They comprise 15% of all primary intracranial tumours and are the most common radiation-induced central nervous system tumour. Sites of occurrence in decreasing frequency are parasagittal convexity, sphenoid wing, planum sphenoidale, supra- or parasellar region, falx, posterior fossa, and spine. Less common sites include the cavernous sinus, cerebellopontine angle, intraventricular region, and orbit.

Meningiomas are typically either iso- or hyperdense on precontrast CT and enhance strongly and homogeneously. They are usually well defined and round in shape. They occasionally demonstrate calcification and cystic degeneration. They may provoke changes in the nearby bone—most often hyperostosis and, much less commonly, erosion. The presence of erosion is suggestive of a malignant lesion such as a metastasis or, very rarely, a malignant meningioma.

Surgical excision results in a permanent cure in the majority of patients with a readily accessible tumour. The meningioma 'en plaque' variant (which resembles pancakes rather than a mass), particularly in the parasellar region or on the lesser wing of the sphenoid, may invade bone and is technically more difficult to excise. This type of tumour may be treated with radiotherapy.

Question 93

This 67-year-old lady presented with a history of increasing confusion and tiredness. Describe the abnormality on this contrast-enhanced CT of the brain (Fig. 93). Suggest a diagnosis.

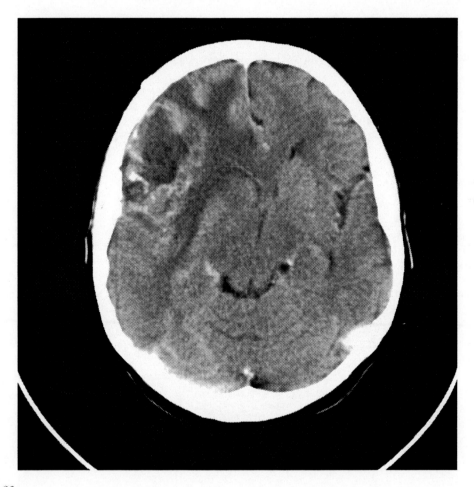

Fig. 93

Answer 93: Primary cerebral malignant tumour

Findings: There is a large irregular heterogeneous mass in the right frontal lobe. Its wall is high density, which may be due to contrast enhancement. There is adjacent low density in the white matter consistent with vasogenic oedema. There is extensive mass effect as seen by the effacement of the right lateral ventricle and the midline shift to the left.

A grade IV astrocytoma (glioblastoma multiforme)

The differential diagnosis for a ring-enhancing cerebral mass is the following:

1   Tumours:
    • Metastasis. More likely in the older age group and if multiple. Most frequently, primary malignancies are bronchus and breast;
    • Primary brain tumour, particularly high-grade gliomas but also lymphoma.
2   Abscess. The wall of the lesion tends to be thinner and more constant in thickness than is the case with necrotic metastases.
3   Vascular lesions:
    • Infarction (may show gyral or serpiginous enhancement), haematomas, and contusion;
    • Resection site;
    • Thrombosed aneurysm.
4   Demyelinating plaques.

Gliomas are the most common primary brain tumours. They are derived from the interstitial tissues of the brain. Most are astrocytomas (80%) but other forms include brainstem glioma and oligodendroglioma.

The astrocytomas are divided into four grades based on histology. The most malignant and common is the grade IV or glioblastoma multiforme. It is more common in older populations, and may arise both *de novo* and from upgrading of lower grade tumours. The appearances shown here are typical. These tumours frequently bleed and demonstrate necrosis and extensive oedema.

Question 94

This 76-year-old man has a long history of low back pain with a more recent increase in symptoms. Describe the abnormalities on the sagittal (Fig. 94a) and axial (Fig. 94b) L5/S1 level, T2-weighted MR of the lumbar spine.

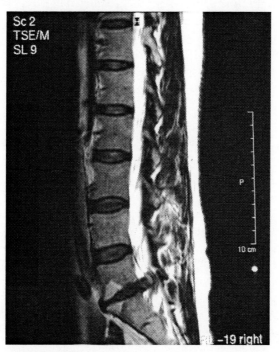

Fig. 94a

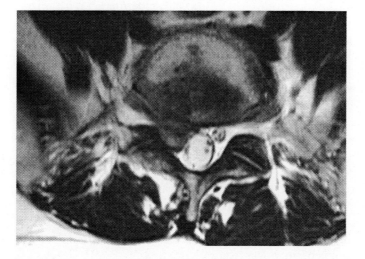

Fig. 94b

Answer 94: L5/S1 disc herniation causing impingement of the right S1 root nerve

Findings: The sagittal image shows loss of the normal high signal of the L5/S1 disc with reduction of the disc height in keeping with degeneration. There is posterior disc herniation into the spinal canal. The axial image (Fig. 94c) shows a prominent right paracentral disc herniation at the L5/S1 disc level resulting in posterior displacement and impingement of the right S1 nerve root (arrow). Note the normal left S1 nerve root (open arrow) and the thecal sac (T).

Degenerative disorders of the spine are extremely common and produce a high burden of morbidity. There are a multitude of changes that can be seen in the different portions of the spine. Disc degeneration is seen initially on MR as the loss of fluid in the nucleus pulposus (desiccation). This is seen as loss of the usual high T2 signal in the centre of the disc.

A *bulge* is defined as extension of disc material up to 3 mm beyond the vertebral endplate for more than 50% of the disc circumference. Disc bulges are usually circumferential and symmetric and are most common at the L5/S1 level. A disc bulge is secondary to laxity of the annulus fibrosis without evidence of a concentric tear. *Disc herniation* is defined as extension of disc material beyond the limits of the intervertebral disc space; this can be focal or broad-based. If less than 25% of the disc circumference is involved, the herniation is termed focal. It is called broad-based if 25–50% of the disc circumference is involved. An *extrusion* is a focal disc herniation with a narrow base of attachment to the original disc, whereas a *pro-trusion* (broad based herniation) has a wide attachment to the underlying disc. A fragment of disc material can become completely separated from the parent disc (termed 'sequestration' or 'free fragment') and can move up or down the spinal canal producing symptoms at levels distant from the original disc. The location of the herniation is described as central, paracentral (right or left of central), intraforaminal, or extraforaminal (lateral).

Root symptoms may be produced by compression in the neuroforamena. The root is named after the superior vertebra. It is also possible for the bulging intervertebral disc to compress the nerve root in the lateral recess. In this case it is the nerve root from the level above that is affected (e.g. a L4/5 disc compressing the L4 nerve root). Surgery may be performed at the wrong level if the radiological anatomy is not precisely defined. Nerve roots may also be compressed in the thecal sac by a central disc bulge. This usually produces symptoms at several levels.

It has been shown that a large number of asymptomatic individuals have disc bulges and protrusions. In symptomatic patients treatment is initially conservative with a large proportion responding. Surgery is reserved for severe symptoms, the presence of neurological deficits, or failed conservative therapy. Failure to relieve symptoms or recurrent symptoms following surgery is known as 'failed back' syndrome. This may be due to scar formation, recurrent disc herniation, arachnoiditis, missed free disc fragments, and surgery at the wrong level. Postoperative MR is useful for distinguishing residual and recurrent disc herniation, which does not show significant contrast enhancement, from scar tissue, which does enhance.

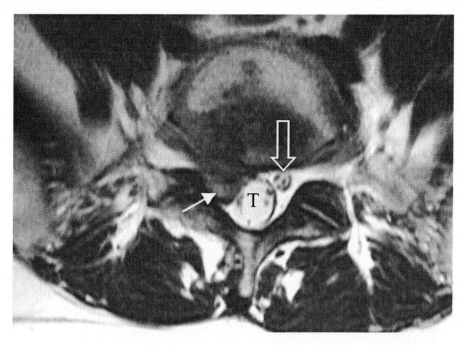

Fig. 94c Axial T2-weighted MR of the lumbar spine at the L5/S1 level showing a right paracentral disc herniation resulting in posterior displacement and impingement of the right S1 nerve root (arrow). Note the normal left S1 nerve root (open arrow) and the thecal sac (T) containing the other sacral nerve roots.

Question 95

This 21-year-old man presented with a 2 day history of worsening scrotal pain. Describe the abnormalities present on the grey-scale (Fig. 95a) and colour Doppler ultrasound images of the left testicle (Fig. 95b). What is the diagnosis?

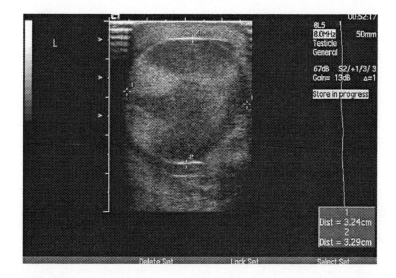

Fig. 95a

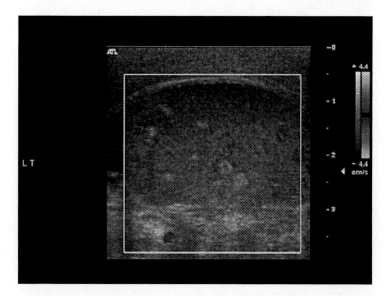

Fig. 95b

Answer 95: *Left testicular infarction due to torsion*

Findings: The grey-scale image (Fig. 95a) shows an enlarged left testicle that has a very heterogeneous echogenicity. The colour flow Doppler image (Fig. 95b) demonstrates no flow in the left testis when compared to the right (not shown). At surgery the left testis was found to be infarcted and an orchidectomy was performed.

Testicular torsion is most commonly seen in puberty (13–16 years) and the neonatal period. There is a 10-fold risk in undescended testes. Torsion outside the neonatal period is intravaginal and is caused by an abnormal tunica vaginalis completely surrounding the testis, epididymis, and the spermatic cord rather than only partially covering the anterior portion of the testis ('bell and clapper' deformity). This allows the testis to turn freely within the vaginalis thus causing compression of the testicular veins and artery. Most 'bell–clapper' anomalies are bilateral making contralateral orchidopexy necessary.

Extravaginal torsion only occurs in the newborn period. Here the torsion occurs at the external ring.

The testis is only viable for 3–6 hours and therefore prompt diagnosis and management is essential. The use of ultrasound (80–90% sensitive) in the diagnosis of torsion is controversial. The most useful sign is loss or reduction in colour Doppler signal of the testis when compared to the contralateral side. Flow in the supplying testicular artery of the spermatic cord should also be sought (sensitivity 44%, specificity 67%). A problem with this approach is that some testes will partially detort, which can lead to normal or increased vascularity in a testis that is still at risk of infarction. However, spontaneous detorsion only occurs in 7%.

Other causes of acute scrotal pain include:

- epididymo-orchitis;
- torsion of testicular appendix;
- strangulated inguinal hernia;
- trauma.

Other rarer causes include testicular neoplasm and abdominal causes including renal colic, pancreatitis, appendicitis, and lumbar radiculopathy.

Question 96

This 64-year-old lady presented with sudden onset severe chest pain and collapse. A contrast-enhanced CT of her chest at the level of the main pulmonary artery was performed (Fig. 96a). What is the diagnosis?

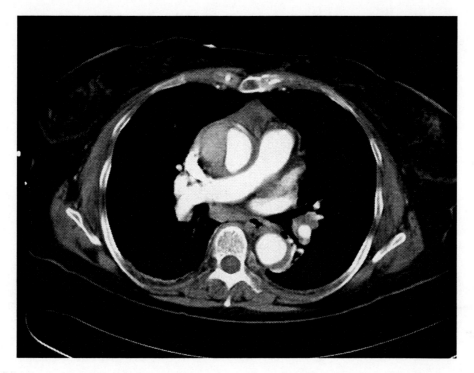

Fig. 96a

Answer 96: Thoracic aorta dissection

Findings: There is a thoracic aortic dissection as demonstrated by a dissection flap in both the ascending and descending aorta (dark line in the lateral portions of the aorta). This is a DeBakey type 1 or Stanford type A. A sagittal CT reformat in another patient shows a dissection flap extending into the abdominal aorta (Fig. 96b).

Aortic dissection is associated with degeneration of the media of the aortic wall. It is associated with hypertension, collagen disorders (Marfan's, Ehlers–Danlos), aortic valve abnormalities (bicuspid valves), collagen vascular disease (relapsing polychondritis), and pregnancy. It is not associated with syphilitic aortitis.

Two classification systems are in common use. The DeBakey classification divides these aortic dissections into:

type 1   involving the whole of the aorta (29–34%);
type 2   only in the ascending aorta (12–21%);
type 3   only in the descending aorta (50%; best prognosis).

The Stanford classification divides them into:

type A   any dissection involving the ascending aorta;
type B   dissections involving only the descending aorta.

Management of dissections involving the ascending aorta and arch is surgical, whilst management of those limited to the descending aorta is medical. On chest radiograph approximately 60% will demonstrate mediastinal widening. Other findings are blurring of the boundaries of the aorta, disparity in the size of the different portions of the aorta, pleural effusion, and inward displacement of any calcification in the wall. This occurs as most of the calcification is in the intima. Complications include retrograde dissection causing aortic valve regurgitation, coronary artery occlusion, and haemopericardium. Occlusion of other major aortic branches occurs in 30% (Fig. 96c). Mortality for an untreated dissection is high and therefore early diagnosis is essential.

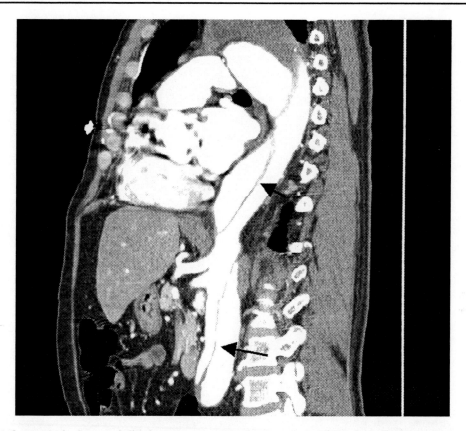

Fig. 96b Sagittal reformatted CT showing an extensive dissection (arrows) involving the thoracic and abdominal aorta.

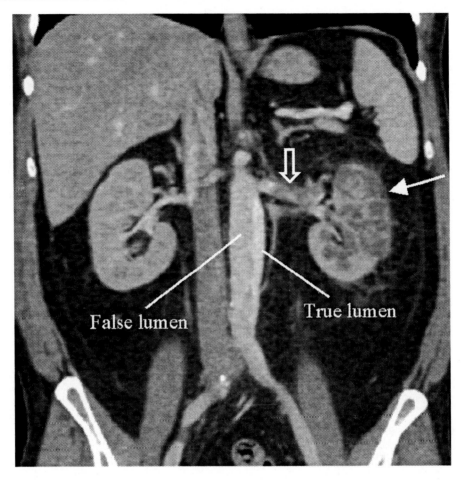

Fig. 96c   Coronal reformatted CT showing a dissection involving the abdominal aorta. Thrombosis of the left renal artery (open arrow), which arises from the false lumen, has resulted in renal infarction (arrow). Note the true and false lumens of the aortic dissection.

Question 97

This 77-year-old man presented with severe abdominal pain and hypotension. A section from an unenhanced CT scan of the abdomen (Fig. 97a) is shown. What is the diagnosis?

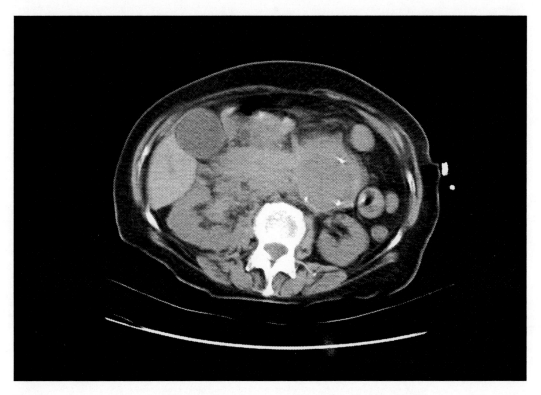

Fig. 97a

Answer 97: Ruptured abdominal aortic aneurysm (AAA)

Findings: Retroperitoneal haemorrhage (arrows, Fig. 97b) extends from the right side of a 6 cm diameter partially calcified abdominal aortic aneurysm (A) to the right kidney (RK), displacing the pancreas (P) anteriorly.

There are several uses of imaging in AAA. In the non-acute setting a CT is helpful for treatment planning. The important issues to determine are whether the aneurysm is supra- or infrarenal, whether the iliac arteries are involved, and whether the left renal vein is retro-aortic or in its normal pre-aortic position. A measurement of the size of the aneurysm can also be made. The normal cross-sectional diameter of the abdominal aorta is taken as less than 3 cm. Ultrasound can be used to monitor the size of the AAA. The incidence of rupture is 10% in an aneurysm less than 4 cm in size, 23% in a 4–5 cm aneurysm, 25% in a 5–7 cm aneurysm, 46% in a 7–10 cm aneurysm, and 60% in aneurysms greater than 10 cm in size.

Increasingly patients are being managed by EVAR (endovascular aneurysm repair). Determining the proximal extent of the aneurysm is particularly important for this procedure because at least a short distance of normal aorta beneath the renal arteries is required to fix the covered stent in place proximally. Measurements of the length and widths of the aneurysm are made. Bespoke stents can be made from these measurements tailored to the individual patient's aneurysm, or stents can be suitably selected from 'off the peg' units. Generally, both common femoral arteries need to be patent to allow this type of repair.

In the acute setting a CT scan may help in the diagnosis of difficult cases of patients with abdominal pain. However, this introduces a delay in a patient who potentially is exsanguinating from a ruptured abdominal aortic aneurysm, and therefore the role of CT is limited. In this setting rupture is demonstrated as blood spilling out into the retroperitoneum particularly over the left psoas muscle. If active bleeding is occurring at the time of a contrast-enhanced CT scan, high-density contrast medium may be seen extravasating at the site of the leak.

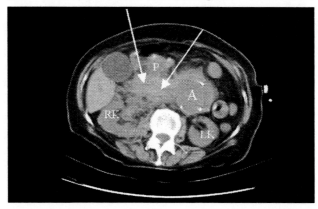

Fig. 97b   Retroperitoneal haemorrhage (arrows) extends from the right side of a 6 cm diameter partially calcified leaking abdominal aortic aneurysm (A) to the right kidney (RK) displacing the pancreas (P) anteriorly. LK, Left kidney.

Question 98

A 58-year-old male with known colonic carcinoma and inguinal lymph node metastases presented with swelling and pain in the right leg. An ultrasound of the right groin area (Fig. 98a) and a colour Doppler ultrasound (Fig. 98b) were performed. What are the findings of interest? What is the diagnosis?

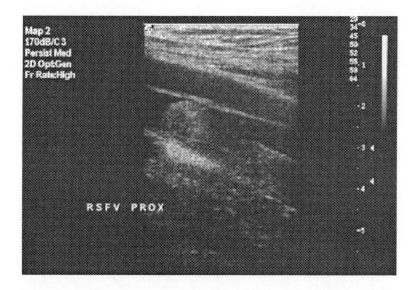

Fig. 98a

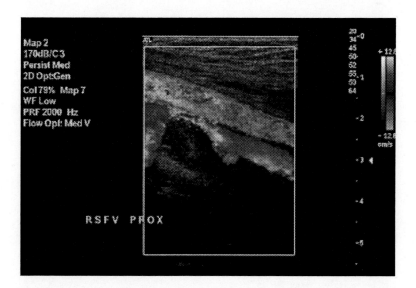

Fig. 98b

Answer 98: Deep venous thrombosis (DVT) of the proximal right superficial femoral vein

Findings: Figure 98a shows an echogenic thrombus in the proximal superficial femoral vein. Figure 98c (Fig. 98b reproduced) shows the corresponding colour Doppler image with flow seen around the deep venous thrombosis (DVT), indicating partial occlusion of the vein.

The other important and the best sign of thrombosis on US examination of the deep venous system, is lack of compressibility of the vein because it is filled with thrombus. The appearance of a thrombus changes with time: initially it is echopoor, becoming isoechoic and then hyperechoic in a matter of weeks. Old thrombi also shrink with time, and their margins become less convex-outwards as the thrombus retracts. The vein may eventually recanalize or partially recanalize.

Ultrasound has replaced contrast venography as the standard imaging investigation for DVT. This has occurred due to cost, operator time, ease of examination and accessibility of Doppler ultrasound, and lack of contrast and radiation exposure. Some radiologists (and clinicians) prefer venography as this allows better evaluation of the calf veins, but there is disagreement about the clinical importance of below knee DVTs and venography can be technically very challenging, especially in patients with swollen legs where venous access is difficult.

Virchow's triad defines the risk categories for DVT. They are:

1 endothelial injury;
2 reduced blood flow;
3 hypercoaguable blood.

Thus the risk factors for DVT include:

- surgery (especially knee and hip), trauma, prolonged immobility;
- malignancy;
- increasing age;
- obesity;
- pregnancy and the oral contraceptive pill;
- smoking;
- activated protein C resistance, protein S and protein C deficiency.

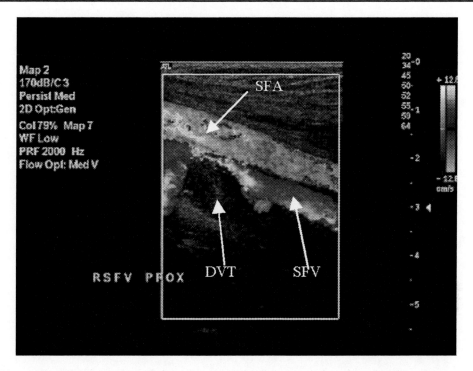

Fig. 98c   Colour Doppler image with flow seen around the deep venous thrombosis (DVT), indicating partial occlusion of the vein. SFA, Superficial femoral artery; SFV, superficial femoral vein.

Question 99

This 28-year-old man presented with a cough that did not resolve with antibiotics. Describe the abnormality on the chest radiograph (Fig. 99a). What would be the next imaging investigation? What is the differential diagnosis?

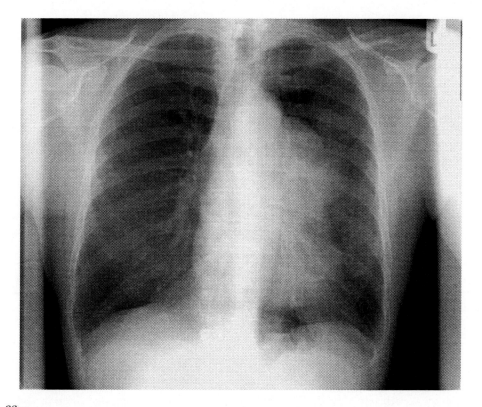

Fig. 99a

Answer 99: Thymoma

Findings: There is a large smooth-edged, lobulated mass, emanating from the left mediastinum, that effaces the left heart border indicating that the mass is in the anterior mediastinum. The lateral border of the descending thoracic aorta is still visible. This means that the mass does not extend into the posterior mediastinum (since the descending thoracic aorta, located in the posterior mediastinum, is still visible, it must be adjacent to air in the lung and not abutting the mass silhouette sign). The left hilar structures can be seen through the mass indicating that the mass does not extend into the middle mediastinum.

The next investigation should be a lateral chest radiograph to confirm the position of the mass in the anterior mediastinum. (The imaging investigation after the lateral chest radiograph should be a CT of the chest.)

Causes of anterior mediastinal masses (commonly remembered as 'the four Ts') are:

- thymoma (or thymic cyst or thymolipoma);
- teratoma (germ cell tumour);
- (retrosternal) thyroid mass (multinodular goitre, thyroid cancer). A thyroid mass must extend up into the neck;
- 'terrible' lymphoma and other causes of lymphadenopathy.

The contrast-enhanced CT (Fig. 99b) confirms that the mass is situated in the anterior mediastinum and shows no significant enhancement. It is homogeneous throughout with no evidence of calcification or necrosis. It extends up to, but does not invade, the great vessels.

The appearances are in keeping with a thymoma or with lymphadenopathy. Thymomas may be associated with myasthenia gravis and, rarely, with aplastic anaemia. One-third are malignant.

Causes of middle mediastinal masses are:

- bronchogenic carcinoma;
- lymphadenopathy (lymphoma, TB, sarcoidosis, metastatic malignant lymph nodes);
- ascending aorta or arch aneurysms or (rarely) aneurysms of other vessels.

Causes of posterior mediastinal masses are:

- hiatus hernia;
- foregut abnormalities (duplication cysts);
- neurogenic tumours.

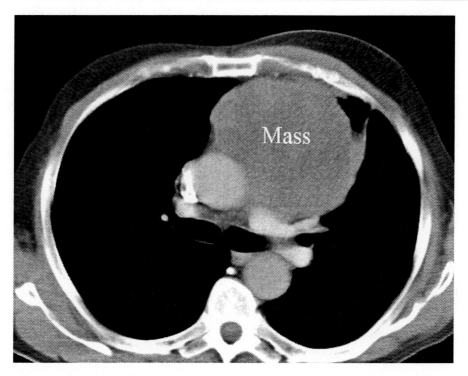

Fig. 99b The contrast-enhanced CT of the chest shows an anterior mediastinal mass and a thymoma was diagnosed histologically.

Question 100

This 58-year-old man presented with right loin pain and haematuria. The enhanced CT of his abdomen is shown (Fig. 100a). Describe the abnormalities. What is the diagnosis?

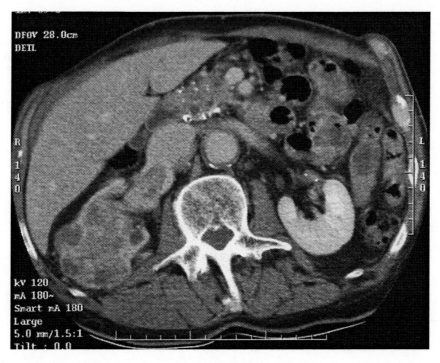

Fig. 100a

Answer 100: Renal cell carcinoma (RCC)

Findings: There is a large, irregular, abnormally enhancing mass replacing the right kidney consistent with a renal cell carcinoma (RCC; Fig. 100b). There is a filling defect in the right renal vein (open arrow, Fig. 100b) consistent with tumour/thrombus. The inferior vena cava (IVC) is patent.

RCC accounts for approximately 3% of visceral cancers and is increasing in incidence. It is seen most frequently in men in their fifties and is associated with smoking, obesity, phenacetin abuse, haemodialysis, renal transplantation, von Hippel–Lindau disease, and tuberous sclerosis. It is a disease that presents late and is resistant to most chemotherapy and to radiotherapy, which is why there has been no significant reduction in mortality in the last 30 years.

Staging is best carried out on CT and MR, both of which are highly accurate. Particular reference must be made to extension of the tumour into the renal (Gerota's) fascia, the renal vein, and the IVC. Lymph node enlargement and distant metastases are also well assessed by these cross-sectional imaging modalities. RCC frequently spreads to lung, liver, bone, the adrenals, and the opposite kidney.

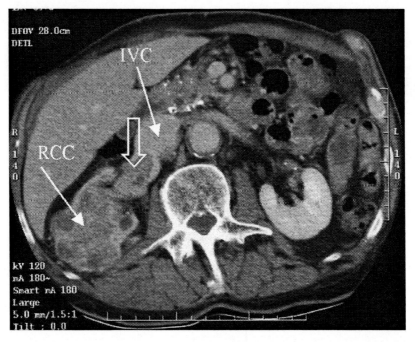

Fig. 100b *CT of the abdomen showing a large, heterogeneously enhancing mass replacing the right kidney consistent with a renal cell carcinoma (RCC). There is a filling defect in the right renal vein (open arrow) consistent with tumour/thrombus. The inferior vena cava (IVC) is patent.*

Question 101

This 64-year-old lady presented with a change in bowel habit. A colonoscopy failed because a segment of sigmoid diverticular disease could not be passed. No abnormality was detected in the visualized colon and rectum. What imaging technique (Fig. 101a) has been performed as an alternative to colonoscopy? What abnormality has been demonstrated?

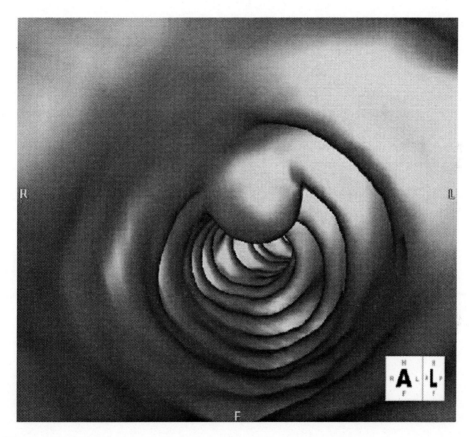

Fig. 101a

Answer 101: CT colonoscopy showing a polyp

Findings: A polyp is present on the endoluminal fly-through virtual colonoscopy. Note the normal colon haustrations.

Over the last few years there has been a great deal of interest and research into virtual colonoscopy originally described in 1994. Using advanced computer software three-dimensional reconstruction of the contiguous volumetric CT data set (virtual colonoscopy, CT colonoscopy) permits a fly-through view of the colonic mucosa similar to that seen endoscopically. Virtual colonoscopy has the advantage of being quicker, better tolerated, safer (no sedation necessary or risk of perforation), and more cost-effective than endoscopy but has the disadvantage of using ionizing radiation. CT is particularly useful in failed conventional colonoscopy/barium enema and in the ill and frail. CT also allows the use of multiplanar reconstructions (Figs 101b and 101c) and images the abdominal and pelvic organs. Bowel cleansing is necessary in both techniques. The CT is performed in the supine and prone positions, to allow optimal visualization of all colon segments, after insufflation of rectal air and an intravenous antispasmodic. The scan is performed during a single breathhold of about 20 seconds. The use of intravenous contrast medium also allows polyps and carcinomas to be distinguished from faeces and bowel folds as well as allowing inspection of the liver for metastases. Faecal tagging and computer-aided diagnosis are promising developments.

Virtual colonoscopy has produced promising results in terms of adenomatous polyp detection with sensitivities and specificities of greater than 95% in the detection of polyps 10 mm in diameter or larger which are similar to those obtained with conventional colonoscopy. For polyps 5–9 mm in size the sensitivity is 70–80% with a specificity of approximately 85%. Further research is continuing to fully assess its impact in terms of use as a screening tool, acceptability, availability, and cost benefit.

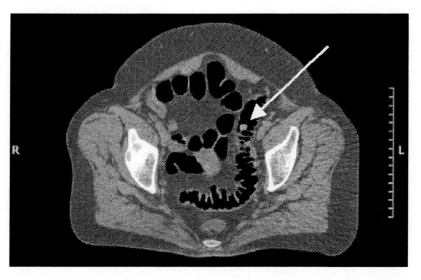

Fig. 101b   Axial CT section demonstrates a 1 cm polyp (arrow) in a segment of sigmoid diverticular disease that could not be passed endoscopically. Therefore the polyp was not detected endoscopically.

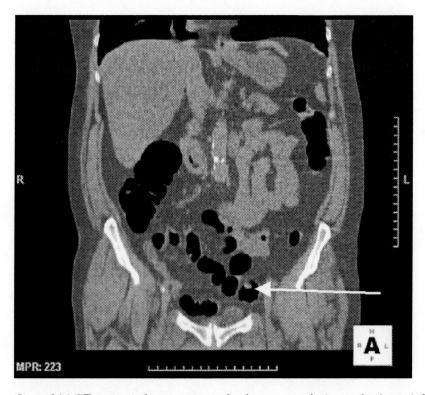

Fig. 101c   Coronal (c) CT section in the same patient also demonstrates the 1 cm polyp (arrow) shown in Fig. 101b.

Bibliography

Armstrong, P., Wilson, A.G., Dee, P., and Hansell, D. (ed.) (2000). *Imaging of diseases of the chest*, 3rd edn. Mosby, St Louis, Missouri.

Dahnert, W. (2003). *Radiology review manual*, 5th edn. Williams and Wilkins, Baltimore.

Gore, R.M. and Levine, M.S. (ed.) (2000). *Textbook of gastrointestinal radiology*, 2nd edn. W.B. Saunders, Philadelphia.

Grainger, R.G., Allison, D.J., Adams, A., and Dixon, A.K. (ed.) (2001). *Diagnostic radiology: a textbook of imaging*, Vols 1–3, 4th edn. Churchill Livingstone, Edinburgh.

Husband, J.E. and Reznek, R.H. (ed.) (1998). *Imaging in oncology*, 1st edn. Isis Medical Media Ltd, Oxford.

Ledingham, J.G.G. and Warrell, D.A. (ed.) (2000). *Concise Oxford textbook of medicine*. Oxford University Press, Oxford.

Meire, H., Cosgrove, D.O., Dewbury, K., and Farrant, P. (ed.) (2001). *Clinical ultrasound: a comprehensive textbook, abdominal and general ultrasound*, Vols 1–2, 2nd edn. Churchill Livingstone, Edinburgh.

Resnick, D. (2002). *Diagnosis of bone and joint disorders*. W.B. Saunders, Philadelphia.

Royal College of Radiologists (1998). *Making the best use of a department of clinical radiology*, 4th edn. Royal College of Radiologists, London.

Shields, T.W. (ed.) (2001). *General thoracic surgery*, 3rd edn. Lea and Febiger, London.

Vahlensieck, M., Genant, H.K., and Reiser, M. (ed.) (2000). *MRI of the musculoskeletal system*. Thieme, Stuttgart.

Index

NB: Page numbers in *italics* refer to tables